SWINE HUSBANDRY.

A Practical Manual for the Breeding, Rearing and Management of Swine,

WITH

SUGGESTIONS AS TO THE PREVENTION AND TREATMENT OF THEIR DISEASES.

By F. D. COBURN.

NEW, REVISED AND ENLARGED EDITION.

ILLUSTRATED

New York:
Orange Judd Company,
1919

PRINTED IN U. S. A.

CONTENTS.

CONTENTS.

PREFACE TO THE THIRD REVISED AND ENLARGED EDITION.

ONCE more has come from its publishers a reminder that the most recent edition of Swine Husbandry has all been sold, and the request that some intended revision shall be speedily prepared, with a view to early supplying the demand which has been continuous since the work was first announced.

With an aim to having it as nearly as may be abreast of the times, various changes have been introduced, and additions made for this issue of facts which were only recently available. The figures in the introductory chapter have been brought down to the latest dates possible. The chapter (somewhat amplified in this edition) of experiments by Prof. E. M. Shelton, at the Kansas State Agricultural College, on "The Effects of Cold upon Fattening Swine," and that by Prof. W. A. Henry, of the Wisconsin Experiment Station, on "Feeding for Fat and Lean," will be found not only especially interesting and instructive, but also the most suggestive recent additions to swine literature. For their arrangement and careful revision especially for this volume, grateful acknowledgment is hereby made. To Mr. Charles B. Murray, editor of the *Cincinnati Price Current*, Hon. L. N. Bonham, and secretaries of the various swine breeders' associations, the author is also indebted for very valuable data furnished.

F. D. COBURN.

KANSAS CITY, KANSAS, 1897.

PREFACE TO FIRST EDITION.

In preparing this work, I have acted upon the belief that no one man, or any half-dozen men, know all there is worth knowing on a subject so extensive and important as that of Swine Husbandry; still, there are many men who know *something* concerning some branch of it, which they have learned by long experience, careful study, and close observation, and who have acquired their knowledge under precisely such conditions and circumstances as to-day surround many other men, who have neither experience nor sound advice to guide them.

It has been less my object to make an original book, filled with fine theories, and the limited experiences of one individual, than to condense in one small volume, from all available sources, the conclusions and ideas of the most practical, successful, observant men who have followed the business in our own time, and in our own country, leaving the reader free to form his own conclusions, and pursue such methods as shall, with the light before him, seem most rational and profitable.

As to the choice of breeds of swine, I have my preferences, which will be found freely expressed elsewhere, but I can fully appreciate the fact, that a breed exactly suited to the wants of farmers in one locality, might not meet the needs of those in other portions of the country, who make pork for different purposes, and under widely different circumstances, and for different markets.

So long as mankind differ about so many other matters, it is idle to expect them to agree upon any one breed of swine, or upon one manner of breeding and feeding as being altogether the best.

Each breed has its champions, and each, in proper hands, under favorable circumstances, with congenial food and climate, has proven itself entirely satisfactory; while animals of the same breed, but with different treatment and surroundings, would have been found in every way unsatisfactory, and discarded for what their owner considered positive knowledge of their worthlessness.

I am confident that each of the leading breeds has its place and its merits, and for this reason I have not undertaken to exalt any one of them over another. One person, by a lucky purchase of animals of a certain breed, and by proper management, attains unusual success, and from that time is satisfied in his own mind, that he possesses a breed incomparably better than any other; at the same time, some other person, with a breed of entirely different characteristics, has been even more successful, and knows, at least to his own satisfaction, that he possesses the one breed worth having, and cares not to be told that some other may also be valuable.

If this book shall serve to encourage the keeping of better swine, in a better, more rational, and consequently more profitable way, my labors will not have been in vain.

To the many correspondents, breeders, and friends, who proffered assistance and encouragement, and to the numerous journals I have quoted—which I have aimed to duly credit—I am under lasting obligations, and any success this effort attains will be largely due to them.

From the Hon. John M. Millikin (present State Treasurer of Ohio), especially, much valuable information has been obtained.

F. D. COBURN.

POMONA, KANSAS, *April*, 1877.

SWINE HUSBANDRY.

CHAPTER I.

INTRODUCTORY TO THE REVISED EDITION—SOME STATISTICS.

The United States Secretary of Agriculture, in his Annual Report, estimated the number of hogs in the United States in 1896 to be, including pigs, 42,842,759, of an average value of $4.35 each, or a total value of $186,529,745; the highest average valuation per head being in Rhode Island, $9.80, and the lowest, in Florida, $2.16. Of the total number, there were, in the fourteen States that may properly be designated as the Mississippi valley, viz., Wisconsin, Illinois, Indiana, Ohio, Kentucky, Tennessee, Mississippi, Minnesota, Iowa, Nebraska, Missouri, Kansas, Arkansas and Louisiana, 26,949,957 head, or nearly 63 per cent. The average value per head ranged from $6.27 in Wisconsin, to $2.53 in Arkansas, the total value being $119,156,111. In the same report, the corn crop in the United States for the year 1895 is figured at 2,151,138,580 bushels, worth $544,985,534, of which the fourteen Mississippi Valley States mentioned above produced 1,691,408,775 bushels, the farm valuation of which, counted at 22.2 cents per bushel, or $375,369,569, represented 78.62 of the total corn crop, and 69 per cent of its value for the entire Union.

It is no doubt safe to say that few persons have any proper conception of the immensity of the swine-producing interest in the United States, or are aware that nearly one-half in numbers and more than one-half in value of all the swine in the world, are reared and fattened in this country. The distribution of the world's supply, according to the most recent available returns, is shown in the table below, which gives the number in the United States in 1896, in the United Kingdom in 1896, British North American Provinces in 1894, and in other countries having 100,000 or more somewhat earlier:

Country	Number	Country	Number
United States	42,842,759	Portugal	720,000
Russia	9,242,997	Belgium	646,375
Germany	12,174,288	Australasia	1,027,714
Austro-Hungary	8,353,339	Denmark	829,131
France	5,860,952	Sweden	682,178
Spain	4,352,000	Holland	543,900
United Kingdom	2,878,801	Argentine Republic	350,000
Switzerland	565,781	Greece	175,000
Italy	1,800,000	Cape Good Hope	228,764
B. N. A. Provinces	1,702,785	Norway	120,737
Roumania	926,124		
		Total	96,023,625

The gradual variation in the number of swine in the United States during the twenty-five years prior to and including 1896, is well shown in the following figures. These are the estimates by the United States Department of Agriculture, of the number in January of each year:

Year	Number	Year	Number	Year	Number
1872	31,796,300	1881	36,227,603	1889	50,301,592
1873	32,632,000	1882	44,122,200	1890	51,602,780
1874	30,860,900	1883	43,270,086	1891	50,625,106
1875	28,062,200	1884	44,200,893	1892	52,398,019
1876	25,726,800	1885	45,142,657	1893	46,094,807
1877	28,077,100	1886	46,092,043	1894	45,206,498
1878	32,262,500	1887	44,612,836	1895	44,165,716
1879	34,766,200	1888	44,346,525	1896	42,842,759
1880	34,034,100				

Mr. Charles B. Murray, editor of the *Cincinnati Price Current,* who is the most prominent authority on figures pertaining to the subject, estimates the number of hogs packed in the United States in the twelve months ending March 1, 1893, 1894, 1895 and 1896, as shown below:

	1895-96.	1894-95.	1893-94.	1892-93.
Packed in the West	15,010,000	16,003,000	11,605,000	12,390,000
Packed at Boston	1,290,000	1,748,000	1,578,000	1,784,000
Other New England packing	677,000	698,000	585,000	649,000
Packed at Buffalo	463,000	475,000	402,000	455,000
Other Eastern packing	173,000	178,000	136,000	128,000
Receipts, N. Y., Phila., Balt.	2,867,000	2,517,000	2,483,000	2,790,000
Total	20,480,000	21,619,000	16,789,000	18,196,000

These figures represent only the organized pork packing of the country, done in cities; and to obtain the aggregate number slaughtered, there should be added those killed by farmers for home consumption and limited neighborhood sale, in weight about two-thirds as much more, and in numbers a somewhat larger proportion.

The exports of live hogs from the United States to foreign countries are reported by the National Bureau of Statistics, for each of the twenty-five years named below (ending June 30th), as follows:

Year	Number	Year	Number	Year	Number
1871	8,770	1880	83,434	1888	23,755
1872	56,110	1881	77,456	1889	45,128
1873	99,720	1882	36,368	1890	91,148
1874	158,581	1883	16,129	1891	95,654
1875	64,979	1884	46,382	1892	31,963
1876	68,044	1885	55,025	1893	27,375
1877	65,107	1886	74,187	1894	1,553
1878	29,284	1887	75,383	1895	7,130
1879	75,129				

The exports of bacon (including sides, hams and shoulders), pork and lard, to foreign countries, as officially reported by the Statistical Bureau, for each of the twenty-five years ending June 30, were:

	Bacon, lbs.	Pork, lbs.	Lard, lbs.	Average Export Value, cts. per lb.	Total value.
1871	71,446,854	39,250,750	80,037,297	12.05	$22,992,023
1872	246,208,143	57,169,518	199,651,660	8.99	45,426,519
1873	395,381,737	64,147,461	230,534,207	8.88	61,274,987
1874	347,405,405	70,482,379	205,527,471	9.38	58,500,639
1875	250,286,549	56,152,331	166,869,393	12.08	57,184,630
1876	327,730,172	54,195,118	168,405,839	12.32	67,837,963
1877	460,057,146	69,671,894	234,741,233	10.64	81,371,491
1878	592,814,351	71,889,255	342,766,254	8.60	86,687,858
1879	732,249,576	84,401,676	326,658,686	6.90	78,738,674
1880	759,773,109	95,949,780	374,979,286	6.89	84,838,242
1881	746,944,545	107,928.086	378,142,496	8.49	104,660,065
1882	468,026,640	80,447,466	250,367,740	10.37	82,852,946
1883	340,258,670	62,116,302	224,718,474	11.32	70,966,268
1884	389,499,368	60,363,313	265,094,719	9.75	69,740,456
1885	400,127,119	72.073,468	283,216,339	8.59	64,883,110
1886	419,788,796	87,267,715	293,728,019	7.13	57,125,408
1887	419,922,955	85,869,367	321,533,746	7.45	61,658,685
1888	375,439,683	58,900,153	297,740,007	8.10	59,299,852
1889	400,224,646	64,133,639	318,242,990	8.52	66,716,097
1890	608,490,956	80,068,331	471,083,598	7.35	85,281,174
1891	599,085,665	82,136,239	498,343,927	7.19	84,908,698
1892	584,776,389	80,714,227	460,045,776	7.56	85,116,566
1893	473,936,329	53,372,366	365,693,501	9.46	84,554,822
1894	503,628,148	64,744,528	447,566,867	9.19	93,433,582
1895	558,044,099	58,266,893	474,895,274	8.22	89,696,768

The quantity and value of lard oil exported in the twenty-five years subsequent to and including 1871, ending June 30, is stated as follows:

Year.	Gallons.	Value.	Value per gal.	Year.	Gallons.	Value.	Value per gal.
1871	147,802	153,850	104.09	1884	712,696	504,218	70.75
1872	533,147	432,483	81.12	1885	916,157	555,426	60.63
1873	388,836	298,751	76.31	1886	973,229	500,011	51.38
1874	252,577	203,317	80.50	1887	975,163	519,274	53.25
1875	146,594	147,384	100.54	1888	930,616	509,514	54.73
1876	146,323	149,156	101.93	1889	861,303	542,897	63.03
1877	347,305	281,551	81.07	1890	1,214,611	663,343	54.61
1878	1,651,648	994,440	60.21	1891	1,092,448	562,986	51.53
1879	1,963,208	1,087,923	52.87	1892	901,575	496,601	55.08
1880	1,507,596	816,447	54.15	1893	486,812	336,613	69.14
1881	836,255	558,576	66.79	1894	681,081	449,571	66.00
1882	506,259	434,124	85.75	1895	553,421	304,093	55.00
1883	379,205	353,184	93.14				

The following table shows the distribution of American hog products by exportation to the principal purchasing countries, and the quantities taken by each, and their value, during the year ending June 30, 1895:

Countries.	* Bacon, lbs.	Pork, lbs.	Lard, lbs.
United Kingdom	436,010,562	14,268,862	184,251,911
France	9 842,048	236,600	34,665,860
Germany	15,137,893	2,149,850	104,121,137
Belgium	40,026,963	258,000	38,163,335
Netherlands	9,631,192	491,282	28,456,561
Denmark	458,019	....	6,952,467
Sweden and Norway	2,618,924	167,900	3,357,535
Spain	60,316	....	70,134
Italy	20,915	....	625,760
Cuba	9,067,529	462,640	30,672,512
Hayti	332,032	13,507,550	3,267,090
Porto Rico	1,079,633	3,285,200	3,414,798
British West Indies	596,378	7,469,033	2,430,443
Mexico	297,599	2,068	1,908,076
Brazil	22,582,582	1,123,292	12,556,491
Colombia	98,902	83,314	1,928,235
Venezuela	680,551	25,200	6,754,790
British Guiana	263,803	2,885,190	395,347
Peru	18,316	15,100	89,851
Quebec, Ont., etc.†	7,124,426	4,757,080	2,139,740
Nova Scotia, etc	66,798	1,208,443	71,112
Newfoundland, etc	203,228	2,020,340	187,081
All Other	1,825,490	3,849,949	8,415,008
Total	558,044,099	58,266,893	474,895,274
Value	$48,736,860	$4,138,400	$36,821,508

* Includes sides, hams and shoulders.

† Includes Manitoba, Northwest Territories and British Columbia.

Below is seen the total number of hogs packed in the West during winter seasons, and cost of hogs per one hundred pounds gross, for fifty years, according to *Cincinnati Price Current* special reports:

Season.	No.	Cost.	Season.	No.	Cost.
1895-96..........	6,815,800	$3.68	1869-70..........	2,635,312	$9.22
1894-95..........	7,191,520	4.28	1868-69..........	2,499,873	8.18
1893-94..........	4,884,082	5.26	1867-68..........	2,781,084	6.36
1892-93..........	4,633,520	6.54	1866-67..........	2,490,791	5.78
1891-92..........	7,761,216	3.91	1865-66..........	1,785,955	9.34
1890-91..........	8,173,126	3.54	1864-65..........	2,422,779	11.46
1889-90..........	6,663,802	3.66	1863-64..........	3,261,105	5.36
1888-89..........	5,483,852	4.99	1862-63..........	4,069,520	3.36
1887-88..........	5,921,181	5.04	1861-62..........	2,893,666	2.42
1886-87..........	6,439,009	4.19	1860-61..........	2,155,702	4.57
1885-86..........	6,298,995	3.66	1859-60..........	2,350,822	4.73
1884-85..........	6,460,240	4.29	1858-59..........	2,465,552	5.02
1883-84..........	5,402,064	5.18	1857-58..........	2,210,778	3.89
1882-83..........	6,132,212	6.28	1856-57..........	1,818,468	4.75
1881-82..........	5,747,760	6.06	1855-56..........	2,489,502	4.60
1880-81..........	6,919,456	4.64	1854-55..........	2,124,404	3.37
1879-80..........	6,950,451	4.18	1853-54..........	2,534,770	3.35
1878-79..........	7,480,648	2.85	1852-53..........	2,201,110	4.81
1877-78..........	6,505,446	3.99	1851-52..........	1,182,846	3.56
1876-77..........	5,101,308	5.74	1850-51..........	1,332,867	3.00
1875-76..........	4,880,135	7.05	1849-50..........	1,652,220	2.13
1874-75..........	5,566,226	6.66	1848-49..........	1,560,000	3.75
1873-74..........	5,466,200	4.34	1847-48..........	1,710,000	2.60
1872-73..........	5,410,314	3.73	1846-47..........	800,000	2.85
1871-72..........	4,831,558	4.12	1845-46..........	900,000	3.90
1870-71..........	3,695,251	5.26	....	....	....

The following table indicates the average gross weights of hogs packed in the West during winter seasons for fifteen years, the average pounds of lard yielded per hog, and their cost per one hundred pounds alive.

Season.	Gross Weight, per hog.	Lbs. of Lard, all kinds.	Cost Alive, per 100 lbs.
1895-96......................	240.71	35.53	$3.68
1894-95......................	232.73	33.62	4.28
1893-94......................	248.20	36.07	5.26
1892-93......................	227.73	31.66	6.54
1891-92......................	247.64	34.69	3.91
1890-91......................	239.75	33.45	3.54
1889-90......................	250.92	36.37	3.66
1888-89......................	263.46	34.76	4.99
1887-88......................	242.30	31.06	5.04
1886-87......................	251.31	33.54	4.19
1885-86......................	258.98	35.22	3.66
1884-85......................	266.51	36.02	4.29
1883-84......................	251.44	33.25	5.18
1882-83......................	267.02	35.43	6.28
1881-82......................	262.70	36.44	6.06

The average live weight of hogs, average cost per one hundred pounds live weight, and percentage yield of lard from those packed at the points named, in the winter seasons of 1894-95 and 1895-96, is shown as follows:

	Average Weight.		Cost, 100 lbs.		Lard percent.	
	1895-96.	1894-95.	1895-96.	1894-95.	1895-6.	1894-95
Chicago	248.59	246.61	$3.81	$4.36	15.59	15.28
Kansas City	243.53	234.29	3.57	4.16	15.02	14.20
South Omaha	268.25	208.95	3.55	4.13	14.62	14.44
St. Louis	224.73	223.61	3.68	4.28	14.25	14.11
Indianapolis	213.60	225.97	3.62	4.34	15.42	14.76
Cincinnati	233.46	235.57	3.71	4.35	15.65	18.57
Milwaukee	243.91	228.22	3.67	4.46	12.55	12.70
Cudahy	239.50	224.00	3.68	4.35	11.48	11.60
Cleveland	190.00	188.00	3.85	4.40	12.70	13.30
St. Paul	225.00	230.00	3.65	4.15	14.22	13.43
Cedar Rapids	244.00	226.00	3.52	4.15	13.93	13.27
Ottumwa	226.00	218.00	3.50	4.15	13.27	13.30
Louisville	224.21	227.91	3.67	4.39	13.70	11.85
Sioux City	264.00	220.00	3.46	4.15	15.15	13.63
Detroit	211.00	215.13	3.80	4.35	13.27	13.94
St. Joseph	265.00	240.00	3.45	4.15	15.09	12.91
Nebraska City	278.00	235.00	3.53	4.15	11.03	13.38
Des Moines	256.00	222.00	3.50	4.09	15.23	14.41
Keokuk	235.00	215.00	3.50	4.19	14.04	13.72
Lincoln	249.00	215.00	3.51	4.00	13.25	11.16
All points	240.71	232.73	3.68	4.28	14.76	14.44

CHAPTER II.

COMPARATIVE VALUE OF THE HOG PRODUCT.

The importance and value to our people of the swine grown in the United States, compared with other kinds of live stock, as shown by official figures, and records that are beyond question, are quite astonishing to those who, for the first time, have them brought to their attention. So long as these animals bring to the coffers of Americans more money than any other single agricultural product, unless it may be wheat or cotton, they are certain to occupy a very high position in the estimation of the producers. Of the money-producing value of swine, as compared with cattle, Hon. John M. Millikin, of Ohio, one of the most experienced and intelligent observers in this direction that our country has ever had, several years ago made some careful estimates, based on authentic data, that reveal what to many will be a condition of affairs not before suspected. Basing his figures on the United States Census for 1870, he says: "The number of cattle then in the country was 23,820,508, and of swine 25,703,813. In the five stock producing States of Kentucky, Ohio, Indiana, Illinois, and Missouri, there were 6,031,819 cattle, and 10,446,198 swine, the excess of the latter over the former being about or upwards of 70 per cent. In view of the above, from which source do the people of the States named derive the largest amount of money per annum?

"The question cannot be answered with entire accuracy, because there are no certain data by which to determine the number or percentage of each kind of animals sold, or the price realized for each head, and yet the result can be closely approximated. Cattle are usually sold at ages varying from three to six years; milch cows and working cattle, which constitute 42 per cent of the entire number, as above stated, generally attain an age exceeding six years before they are sold to go out of the country. As cattle, including all classes, have to arrive at an age above three years, it is safe to say there are not more than one-fourth the number enumerated sold in each year. With hogs it is quite different. They are shipped off at an average age of about fifteen months, and it is therefore fair to assume that at least four-fifths of the hogs enumerated in 1870 were sold within a year from the time of enumeration.

"Upon these data let us make a calculation:

"Upon the hypothesis stated, that *one-fourth* of the cattle enumerated would be sold during the year, there would be sold 1,507,954. Estimating the average value of the same as consumed upon the farm, or sold and shipped at $30 per head, they would amount to the sum of $45,238,620. The total number of hogs in the above States being 10,446,198, *four-fifths* of which were sold during the year, would make the number sold 8,356,952. Estimating these on the farm, when sold or consumed, at the moderate price of $8 per head, the total value is $66,955,672, making the excess received per annum for hogs, over amount received for cattle, in the five States named, $21,717,052.

"I am aware that the above showing will be satisfactory to only a few persons, and that it will be sharply criticised by others. I have made it upon the above data, with a view to seeing what the result would be, and not with a view of depreciating the value and advantages of raising cattle, nor of unduly exalting the business of raising pork."

At the present time, Chicago is considered the greatest live stock market in the world, and the statistics of the live stock trade there, for the year 1873, disclose the startling fact that swine not only brought more money into the pockets of the people than any other description of live stock, *but more than all other kinds together*, as may be seen by an examination of the following table of actual receipts and actual sales in the open market:

	Receipts.	*Sales.*
Cattle	761,428	$35,264,260
Sheep	291,734	875,000
Horses	20,289	2,028,902
Hogs	4,337,750	53,153,000

From these figures, it is seen that the value of the hogs marketed there, exceeded that of all other live stock by nearly $15,000,000, and this does not include any part of the value of the *dressed* hogs, lard, barrelled pork, and cut meats received, the cash value of which amounted to $8,444,494, in the same period, making a total value of $61,597,494.

Chicago also boasts of being the leading grain market of the world, and during the same year (1873), her trade was a prosperous one, the receipts aggregating 10,000,000 bushels more than in the previous year, and the estimated value of this vast quantity was $63,500,000, scarcely $2,000,000 more than the value of the hogs and hog products handled in the same market in that year.

The value of the hog product exported in 1872 from the United States, exceeded $45,000,000, of which England alone took $22,247,167,—more than the entire exportation of cattle products for the same year.

With our fertile, and seemingly inexhaustible soils, both upon the broad prairies and countless creek and river bottoms, the great staple crop is, and ever will be, Indian corn—the grain above all others best adapted to the production of pork; and it is by and through these enormous corn crops that we do and can hold the pork markets of the world at command.

Those who prepare for pork-making with well defined

plans, and pursue them with system and regularity, keeping none but the best breeds and their crosses, can be quite certain of realizing more satisfactory prices for their corn, taking the seasons together, than by selling it at ruling prices, even at their own doors; while if hauled from home, its cost is increased in proportion to the distance, from five to fifteen cents per bushel.

To illustrate the importance of raising the better grades of hogs, we will use some figures from a circular issued by the "Cincinnati Merchants' Exchange" a few years since, which says: "Whole number of hogs packed during the past season, at the principal points in the United States, was 4,782,403; aggregate weight, 1,349,630,955 pounds, or an average weight of 282¹|₄ pounds. The total amount of money paid for same was $55,818,711."—If well bred, well fed, well cared for, and properly fattened, they should have averaged one hundred pounds more per head, adding to the aggregate weight 478,240,300 pounds, which, at four cents per pound, would have added to the wealth of the producers, in a single year, the snug sum of $19,129,-612. Truly no insignificant increase of one year's receipts, and on the same basis amounting in twenty years to $382,592,240—money enough to lift the mortgages from the farms of a large number of worthy gentlemen who think that *one hog is just as good as another.*

BREEDS OF SWINE

THEIR CHARACTERISTICS AND WORTH.

CHAPTER III.

THE POLAND-CHINAS.

Probably no questions have been more frequently propounded to agricultural and live stock journals, than those as to the origin, history and correct name of the large spotted hogs, exceedingly popular in the Western States, and which are called, by different breeders, and in different localities, by a great diversity of names. Among the names which have been given them, are: "Magie," "Butler County," "Warren County," "Miami Valley," "Poland," "Poland and China," "Great Western," "Shaker," "Union Village," "Dick's Creek," "Gregory's Creek," "Moore," and others; and inquiries are frequent as to their characteristics, and if all the hogs thus named are not the same breed, which is best? The wranglings and discussions, by the breeders and friends of the different strains of these hogs, as to their origin, the most suitable and expressive name for the breed, and who should have most credit for efforts to perfect and bring them into popular favor, would, if published, fill volumes. The following, prepared by Hon. L. N. Bonham, who has for many years been not only a citizen of Butler county, but a breeder of these hogs, and who has made them and their history a long study, was adopted in 1887, by the National Swine Breeders' Association, as the official history of the breed, and hence it is given here as the accepted version, in lieu of what has before been published on this great and foremost family of pork makers:

The Poland-China hog originated in the Miami valley, and it is nowhere apparent that it originated from the purpose or work of any one individual. The conditions of soil, climate, produce, and markets of that region, all favored the business

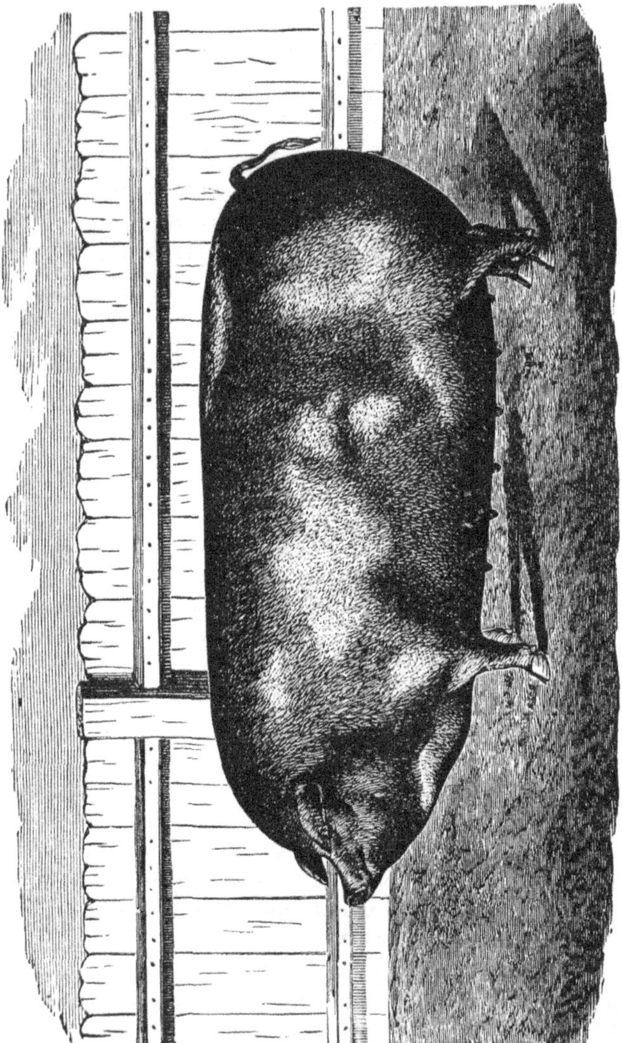

Fig. 1.—POLAND-CHINA SOW.

of swine growing, and, as a result, early in the history of Ohio Cincinnati became, for a time, the greatest pork-packing center in the world, and made pork producing the most profitable feature of farming in the surrounding country.

The farmers of Kentucky and Ohio were deeply interested in the common effort to meet the demands of the market, and secure the best possible rewards for their labor and enterprise. Before the advent of improved roads, canals and railways, the concentration of farm products into animals that could be driven to market, induced a general improvement of not only the swine, but the cattle also, of that region. Under the common law of selection, as well as by importation of improved breeds, by the peculiarly favorable conditions of climate, feed and water, by the influence of trade and fashion, the Poland-China breed of swine originated and developed from the common hog of the Miami valley, until it has become the leading breed of the State and many parts of the country.

It is greatly to be regretted that in the earliest history of this breed, we had not, in Ohio and in the West, such facilities for making a record of the work done and means employed by the farmers of the Miami valley, as we now have in the numerous and able stock journals and agricultural papers of this day.

Prior to 1839 there was no paper in the West specially interested in agriculture or live-stock matters. Hence most of the earliest history of the breed, and of swine raising in the West prior to that date, is purely traditional. Happily, however, about the time the interest in pork growing became the leading feature of agriculture in the Miami valley, the *Western Farmer* was started in Cincinnati, in September, 1839. Its editor, Thomas Affleck, was a man of intelligence and a lover of stock. Associated with him was Charles Foster, who was skillful with his pencil as well as with his pen, and left many well executed cuts and descriptions of animals of southern Ohio and northern Kentucky. The written testimony of these two men may be accepted as the most accurate and valuable of any now available.

The history of the English breeds has been better preserved in the writings of Prof. Low, and earlier English writers. That of the Berkshires is, perhaps, best known of any existing breeds. It is valuable as a help to show how breeds originated. The history of these two best known breeds illustrates forcibly a principle in breeding announced by Prof. Brewer, of New

Haven. It is this: "A breed of animals is never made by crossing two and only two distinct breeds, and preserving the better qualities of both. I am not aware," he says, "that there is any such case on record, among all the countless breeds of our domestic animals. But new breeds are often made of several original breeds by a selection from the mongrel progeny."

The evolution of the Berkshire from the old English hog, the Chinese, the Neapolitan, the Siamese, illustrates this principle, though it has occupied nearly a century of time and study of many indefatigable breeders. Its history is full of interest to all breeders of swine, because it is better understood, being more fully recorded in the current writings of this epoch than that of any other breed of swine. Now, as this breed is so important a factor in the early history of swine breeding in the Miami valley, we may first consider it, to better understand the part played by the several breeds employed in the make-up of the one breed, which, following the law of "survival of the fittest," has survived and superseded all the others, and has become the chief in the counties and State where it had its origin.

THE BERKSHIRE ELEMENT.

By noting characteristics of the several breeds employed in the early formation of the Berkshire breed, one may see why they were used, and where the lop ears, sandy or reddish-brown color, spotted with black, described by Prof. Low in 1842, came from. Then, by following along down a quarter of a century, one will see how, by selection, these undesired features were eliminated, and how, by judicious crossing and selection, have been substituted the erect ear, the solid black color, artistically relieved by the clean white on the face and feet and tip of the tail.

No artist's brush could place the colors more deftly and in more complete harmony. The art of the breeder is further handsomely illustrated in the molding of the approved form, the graceful outline, and in securing a harmony of colors now accepted as that of the ideal standard Berkshire. But this was reached only by persistent and long-continued selection and use of crosses intended to eliminate or correct the undesirable characteristics of the early specimens of this noted breed. A. B. Allen says that in 1841, aged men in Berkshire, England, told him that the breed had been known by them from earliest childhood, and yet he and they were still using Siamese crosses—so persistent were the original colors and traits and tendencies to reversion to the hateful characteristics of the old English hog, such as slow feeding, coarseness of ear, hair and form, and the mixed, uncertain colors. Prof. Low tells of the use of the Chinese boars as late as 1842, to refine and improve the feeding quality of this long-known breed.

MONGRELS, OR MIXED BREEDS.

The Bedfords, or Woburns, are spoken of in the *Genesee Farmer* of 1838, as having strenuous advocates in Massachusetts and near Baltimore. In Bedfordshire, England, the Duke of Bedford, who was a successful breeder of Berkshires, is spoken of as an advocate of the Bedfords as a most prolific breed.

In Massachusetts, the name of Woburn was given the breed. Youatt says of them (p. 96): "Some admirable pigs were sent to the great cattle shows of London. They were crosses of various kinds, in which it appeared to us the Suffolk strain was prevalent." Affleck (p. 86), in his chapter on hogs in Ohio and Kentucky, says: "The variation in the character of the half dozen different sorts of Bedfords is also great in size, color and form." He believes those in America were descended from an importation by a Mr. Parkinson, an Englishman, who lived near Baltimore some eighty odd years ago. These were most probably a mongrel from use of Berkshire and Sussex hogs. As bred in Kentucky and Ohio in 1840, Mr. Affleck says: "They vary a good deal in appearance. The head, neck and ears are fine, the latter somewhat rounded and leaning forward and outward; the shoulder generally good, though from close breeding there is a sinking back of the shoulder in a majority of them; the back otherwise remarkably fine, slightly arched, very broad, the ribs coming finely out and supporting the belly better than is common in any other breed; the loins slender, but high above the shoulders to a very great degree; the rump drooping rather suddenly; the ham large, but not as thick and round as it might be; twist fair; the flank in some good, in others badly tucked; the legs generally so good as to resemble those of a deer much more than of a hog; the bones stout and, though large, not too much for an animal of their size, which is equal to 500 or 600 pounds at eighteen months or two years, with good keep;

the skin good and the handling very fine; the hair long, coarse and harsh; said to fatten kindly at any age and upon a less amount of food than any others." The celebrated Banter pigs were of this breed, and fed against a pair of imported Berkshires, "beat them a long way."

As to color, "some were white and some were sandy, with numerous large black spots." The same writer says of the improved Berkshire of 1840, he fully believes "they will surpass the Woburns on similar keep." He says: "The improved Berkshire more nearly approaches the *ne plus ultra* of a perfect animal of this kind than any other. His form is perfect; his legs are, however, too frequently faulty, though by no means always so."

The Berkshire was first introduced into the Miami valley in 1835, by Mr. Munson Beach and Mr. John Reed, from Albany, N. Y., the former bringing a boar, Dick Johnson, and the latter a sow, Superior.

BYFIELDS.

In 1838, the *Genesee Farmer* speaks of a formidable rival to the Bedfords as having arisen in the eastern part of Massachusetts. Essex county claims the honor of originating it as follows: "A farmer in Byfield found, accidentally, in the market, a pig of remarkable appearance, and this laid him the foundation of the breed known as the Byfield breed."

Mr. Affleck described them as he found them in Warren and Butler counties, Ohio, in 1842, where then they were highly esteemed as a cross with the Russian. He says: "Byfields are of great size, white, with heavy lopped ears, flat-sided, but of great length, and others that are beautifully white, their ears small, pointing to their nose, broad back, deep chest, large jowl, short nose, dished face and thin hair." (P. 86, Affleck.) Different grade crosses of these and Russian, and again with the Chinas, have produced the large hog known as the Warren County hog.

THE IRISH GRAZIER.

In 1839, three Irish pigs were brought to Cincinnati by the father of W. W. Greer, of Oxford, Ohio. These pigs were brought, as thousands of others have been before, to America by emigrants from all parts of the world. Mr. Greer, Sr., lived near the seacoast, where they raised vast quantities of potatoes, on which the hogs were raised and fattened. Martin (p. 98) says of Irish pigs: "The plan of fattening on potatoes is not calculated to do justice to the most approved breeds." He further says (p. 98): "Latterly the introduction of some of our best breeds (from England) with which to cross the old Irish swine, had been attended with decided success, although there is room for further improvement. Berkshire, Suffolk, Yorkshire and some Chinese boars and sows have been introduced " Thus we see that the so-called Irish Grazier imported into Ohio was a mongrel. These Greer pigs went into the hands of William Neff, a pork packer of Cincinnati, with whom Mr. Greer was employed in cutting pork the first winter of his residence in Ohio.

Mr. Neff also imported other Irish pigs and sent them into Warren County, where their impress on the swine of that region was marked and favorable.

Mr. Affleck, speaking of the boar, Poppet, imported by Wm. Neff, said: "He would weigh about 450 or 500 pounds when matured, and is a very finely formed animal." Some of that importation and their descendants carry their ears pricked; they have fine length, a splendid barrel, good legs and very fair hams. The hair is scant, though fine, and the skin unpleasantly scurfy but handling well. The cross of the Berkshire boar and Irish sow was called Bettys, and was considered, by many, better stock than either. In this connection, Mr. Affleck said, in 1842: "The Berkshires, Woburns and the Irish Graziers seem to us the most likely to be of most use, and are certainly those attracting most attention at this time" (1842).

In the *Western Stock Journal* of 1870, published by J. H. Sanders & Co., at Sigourney, Iowa, T. J. Conover said: "The Irish Grazier is white, with a few spots of black; upright ears, light jowl, fine coating, and would fatten at any age. They are the stock of hogs that gave the Poland-Chinas their fine coating and symmetrical form." He also said: "John Harkrader took an interest in the Irish Grazier and commenced an improvement on that breed."

THE RUSSIAN HOG.

Of this breed, Cuthbert Johnson, in his Cyclopedia of Rural Affairs, after describing the several fresh breeds of swine, speaks of "other European breeds." Among these he names the Polish and Russian breed as one and the same, and describes it as being "generally small, and of a reddish or yellowish color." Albert D. Thaer, of Germany, in his great work, The Principles of Agriculture, 1810-12, in enumerating and describing the breeds of swine in North Germany, says: "The breeds of swine best known in North Germany, but nevertheless crossed in various ways, are the following: Moldavian, Wallachian and Bothnian pigs, distinguished by great size, dark gray color and very large ears.

"The next class named is the Polish, or, more properly speaking, Podolian pigs, also very large, but of a yellowish color, and having a broad brown stripe along the spine. These two races furnish very large pigs for fattening, but they require a proportionately large quantity of food; besides, they are not very productive; the sows seldom have more than three, four or five young ones at a birth."

We are all well aware that what Thaer has here said of this Polish or Podolian pig of North Germany has been the reliance of some who have tried to argue the Russian hog out of existence. Though the two tawny breeds agree in the stripe down the back, Thaer says: "The Polish breed seldom has more than three or four or five young ones at a litter," while it is notorious that the Reds and their English ancestors are most prolific. It is not probable that they are of similar origin. That there was a large white breed, known by the farmers of Ohio as much as seventy-five years ago as the Russian hog, there is abundance of living and written testimony. James E. Letton, of Millersburg, Ky., in 1840, wrote the following description of them: "Their color is generally white, with long, coarse hair; head long and coarsely featured; their ears are not so broad as the common variety of the country, yet longer and narrower, and come regularly to a point, projecting forward, and they do not appear to have so much command of them as other breeds; they have fine length and hight, their bone is large and fine; they stand well upon their pastern joints and trackers; quite industrious; they are thick through the shoulders, indifferently ribbed (or suddenly inclined down); their plate or kidney bone rather narrow and ovaling than otherwise; hams pretty good, though not so good as the Irish, the Bedford or the Berkshire. Yet preferable as is the variety, they do not grade so well as many others; they want more time to bring them into market than the above breeds. Give them from eighteen to twenty months' age, they will make very large hogs; they are quite prolific, their usual number being from nine to twelve pigs a litter. I have found their cross with the above-named breeds to be a valuable acquisition to their grazing, aptitude to fatten and rapid growth at the same time." That this Russian hog was extensively used as one of the earliest crosses for the improvement of the swine of Ohio and Kentucky, is evident from extant writings and living testimony.

In no other description of breeds can we find the counterpart of that back and loin which has cost us so much time and care to correct. Mr. Letton well described it as "indifferently ribbed, or suddenly inclining down, their plate or kidney bone rather narrow and ovaling than otherwise."

The old Harkrader sow had this Russian back, as well as the color, the large, fine bone, and the strong, short pasterns and trackers. How this hog came to the Miami valley and Kentucky is not known. His source and coming are indefinable, but that this so-called Russian hog was highly esteemed as one of the first crosses to improve the common hog of the country, there can be no question. As to the color, Mr. Letton says they were "generally white."

T. J. Conover said, in 1870: "The Russian hog was sandy and black, with white," but, like hogs generally of that date, their color seems not to have been clearly defined.

THE CHINA.

The breed which did the most for the improvement of the hogs of the Miami valley, as they did for the improvement of swine in England, is the China. The first introduction of this breed in Ohio was in 1816, by the Shakers of Union Village. They were called the "Big China hogs." They were bought in Philadelphia by John Wallace, trustee of the Shaker society near Lebanon. There was one boar and three sows. One sow had some sandy spots on her, in which appeared some small black spots. The boar and other sows were white. By their use on the mongrels by the Russian, Byfield and common hogs, came the Miami Valley hog. That this Shaker importation of Chinas was pure China stock, there is reason to doubt. Nevertheless, they impressed, in a wonderful degree, their offspring with a quicker feeding quality, that seemed to be the leading idea in the improvement of that period.

There are frequent allusions to China hogs and their value, by writers in the *Genesee Farmer*, *The Cultivator* and *Western Farmer*, prior to 1842. They were used and esteemed in the East and West, and made their impress on all breeds with which they were crossed. The use of the China has been beneficial in correcting coarseness of form, in quieting the restless disposition, and increasing the tendency to fatten at any age, and refine the texture and quality of flesh.

THE RED HOG, CALLED "POLAND."

There was another element that we cannot omit, which seems not only to have been the very apple of discord among some of our friends, but its impress among the hogs of Ohio and the West is almost as marked as that of the noted Tamworth boar on English breeds. Their color and vigorous growth seemed to attach themselves most persistently to their posterity, and were potent on all crosses. Whether they could be called a distinct breed we will not here discuss. Affleck and Millikin claim not, but that one Asher, of Chester, Butler county, Ohio, a native of Poland, had red hogs which he claimed to have imported from England, there is strong proof. There was frequent allusion to them in the writings of that day, and to the name Poland given to hogs of their type after 1838. We have a letter from B. G. Schenck, of Franklin, Ohio, in answer to inquiry by L. N. Bonham. He says: "I remember once to have spoken of the red hogs and pigs I saw when a boy, at an old Polander's down near Chester. I remember to have gone with my father to this Pole's to see those red pigs, and I remember now just how they looked. They were of a bright, sandy color, with small black specks all over them. They resembled, in make, according to my recollection of the pigs I saw there, and those raised from the pair my father bought at that time, the Berkshire of to-day, except that they were a little deeper in the body, had a flatter rib, and were shorter in the legs. I remember the Polander telling my father that they were the sandy Berkshires, of England, and that he had imported them. I remember the old imported sow and a yearling sow, a pig of hers. They both had litters of pigs at the time. My father crossed them with his hogs, and for years after there would be a pig with the features of the Polander's hogs. I still think that the name Poland, in our Poland-China hogs, came from this old Polander."

Here we have an element that has made a lasting impression on the hogs of the valley and the whole country. The sandy or reddish color is one that has characterized so many of the breeds in their early history, that it has wonderful staying qualities. It never has been a popular color. The early English breeders did not fancy or seek to perpetuate it, nor have

American breeders. Yet in the early history of swine in America, when color counted but little and growth and feeding qualities much, the law of selection did not then exclude animals of sandy markings as it now does, since fashion makes the old markings unfashionable.

That the law of selection, regardless of color, produces profitable hogs, we know. The record of weights made in fattening establishments of an earlier day will make this clear. The books of Wren & Schaffer, of Middletown, Ohio, show that they packed, in 1879, a lot of thirty-eight Poland-China hogs, averaging six hundred and thirteen pounds gross at twenty-one months old, all fattened by one man in Butler county. From a table at hand we quote gross weights of six hundred and twenty-five raised in Butler county, Ohio, and sold to packers in 1870:

One lot of 80 averaged	574 pounds.
One lot of 40 averaged	516 pounds.
One lot of 38 averaged	570 pounds.
One lot of 48 averaged	513 pounds.
One lot of 42 averaged	517 pounds.
One lot of 30 averaged	504 pounds.
One lot of 20 averaged	501 pounds.
One lot of 45 averaged	536 pounds.
One lot of 75 averaged	493 pounds.
One lot of 60 averaged	490 pounds.
One lot of 40 averaged	713 pounds.
One lot of 12 averaged	773 pounds.

To show that this breed had, in 1870, attained unsurpassed excellence in their readiness to fatten at any age, and their rapid growth, we quote the weights of two lots of pigs fattened when eleven months old:

One lot of 30 averaged, gross	384 pounds.
One lot of 10 averaged, gross	410 pounds.
One lot of 38, older, averaged, net	528.89 pounds.
One lot of 2, older, averaged, gross	719 pounds.

The net average of this last forty pigs was five hundred and thirty-eight pounds.

Such a record shows not only skillful breeding, but rare skill in handling and feeding. It tells, too, of the superior natural advantages of a region where such a breed should be originated and produced by an intelligent and persistent application of the law of selection.

Discussions by the Press and by individuals for nearly a half century, have been the cause of searching and thorough investigation into the matters connected with their early history, the time and manner in which the first crosses were made, and upon what foundation, together with the later crosses and manner of breeding, which combine to make them the leading and favorite breed in many sections famous for the value, size, and quality of their hogs. Owing to the great interest manifested on these points, we have given them much careful study and examination, for the purpose of getting at the bottom facts for the public benefit; but it seems well-nigh impossible to harmonize the conflicting statements of those who ought to be best informed, or to expect the champions of the various views to be pleased with such conclusions as do not accord with their own.

On many points, all who have studied the question closely agree, and on others (of perhaps minor importance to the public) some of the disputants are as far apart as the poles, but we believe none dispute that the main crosses towards its formation as a definite and distinct breed were made in that part of southwestern Ohio lying between the Big Miami and Little Miami rivers, mainly the counties of Butler and Warren, during the years from 1835 to 1840. It is also generally conceded that the groundwork was stock locally known as "Warren County" hogs, which were the result of crossing together the Berkshire, "Byfield," the "Russia," the "Big China," and perhaps the "Bedford" breeds, all large, coarse hogs and slow to grow and fatten, except the "Big Chinas," which possessed the very opposite qualities.

Hon. John M. Millikin, who lived in Butler county well-nigh seventy years, forty-five of which he was a farmer, paid special attention to searching out the history of this breed, its material and makers, and his statement to the author was this:

"The truth is, no one man can say he had more to do in the formation of this breed than another. It was the result of the labors of many. It grew out of the introduction of the China hogs by the Shakers of Union Village, the crossing with the Russia and Byfield, and the subsequent crossing with the Berkshires, and then with the Irish Graziers. After 1841, or 1842, these breeds ceased to exist in either Butler or Warren counties, and (in 1877) have had nothing to do whatever with this breed for the last thirty-four years."

Controversies as to the precise crosses, and by whom and under what particular circumstances they were made fifty years ago, to form the breed now known as Poland-Chinas, may interest a few; but what is vastly more important to millions of people, is the fact that there has been produced a race of swine, now bearing that name, that very many severely practical and intelligent men consider the best pork-packing machines known,—in fact, nearer what the farmers of the great central, corn-producing West need, than any other single breed in existence.

Their size, color, hardiness, docility and good feeding qualities make them favorites when purely bred, and where more fineness of contour, quicker maturity, and a little less size is demanded, we are satisfied the sows bred to Berkshire boars produce the best feeding and farm hogs in the world.

CHAPTER IV.

THE CHESTER WHITES.

Knowing Mr. Thomas Wood, of Chester county, Pennsylvania, to be one of the oldest and most reliable breeders of the Chester Whites, and familiar with them from the beginning, we applied to him as a source of reliable information as to their origin, early history, breeding, etc.

He writes : "The Chester County White hog is a native of Chester county, Pennsylvania, where the breed originated. The first impulse to the improvement of swine in this county was induced by the introduction of a pair of very fine white pigs, brought from Bedfordshire, England, by Captain James Jeffries, of this county, and put upon his farm on the Brandywine Creek, near West Chester, the county seat, in the year 1818. Some of our more enterprising farmers, seeing these finely-bred pigs, were induced to commence an improvement of their swine by a cross of these, their progeny, and others of the best hogs of the county, and by continuing a careful selection and judicious crossing for many years, have produced the Chester White of to-day, a most desirable, well-formed, good-sized, easily-fattened, and perhaps the best bacon hog for the general farmer in this or any other country.

"I have been paying considerable attention to the improvement of the Chester Whites for over forty years, and was among the first to disseminate the stock over the United States. I have shown them at numerous agricultural exhibitions ; at the exhibition of the United States Agricultural Society, held at Philadelphia, in 1856, I received the Society's diploma for the best pigs ; at the United States Agricultural Fair, held at Richmond, Va., in 1858, I exhibited Chester Whites, and they took all the highest prizes offered by the Society ; I also exhibited

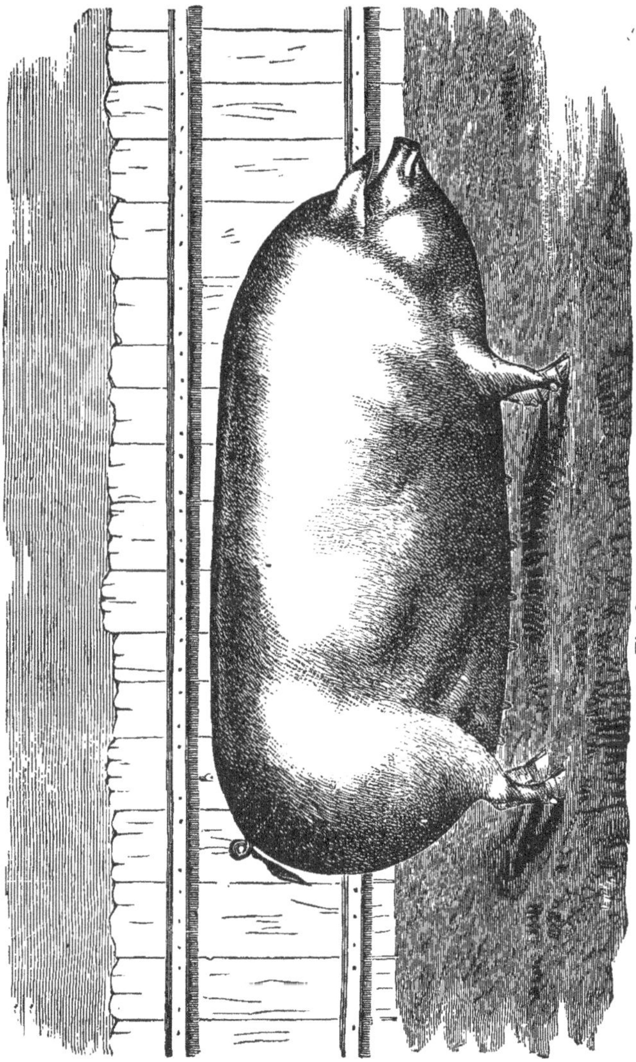

Fig. 2.—CHESTER WHITE SCW.

them at the joint fair of the States of Virginia and North Carolina, held at Petersburg, taking not only the highest premium awarded, but also the sweepstakes premium for the best sow, with considerable competition with other breeds at all these exhibitions.

"The Chester Whites have been successfully exhibited at several fairs of the Maryland Agricultural Society; also at nearly every fair held by the Pennsylvania State Society, as well as by many County Societies, in competition with most other breeds, while in many other States they have successfully competed with all the foreign and home-made breeds.

"Some thirty years ago, the Berkshires were introduced into Chester county, where some of our farmers tried and kept them very nice, and exhibited them at the agricultural fairs; but they did not seem to take well with our farmers at that time, and were displaced by Chesters.

"A few years later the little Suffolks, that were making quite a stir in the hog line in New England, were introduced into our county, and afterwards the Essex, but neither breed flourished here, and the Chesters quietly superseded them.

"I tried them all, but found none of them superior to our own breed. Some of the Chesters had been crossed with the black breeds, and it took our farmers eight or ten years to get rid of their spotted hogs, which was finally pretty well accomplished, and the Chesters again held sway over the county, and hundreds and thousands of them were shipped to different parts of the United States, Canada, and the West Indies. During this time, many unprincipled parties shipped any kind of a white pig they could pick up in the county, which they would call genuine Chesters; this lowered the popularity of the breed wherever such pigs were sent. This caused a great falling off in the demand for our pigs, and again the Berkshires were introduced into this and adjoining counties, they having, in the thirty years since their first introduction, been much improved, and being popular abroad, some of our swine breeders procured them to breed for shipping purposes, and, as every generation must try the different kinds of stock for themselves, many farmers bought the Berkshires to see if they possessed any advantages over the Chester Whites, it being said that their hams were not so fat, and would sell more readily in market. After many years of trial, many farmers said that the white hogs were best adapted to their wants.

"The Yorkshires have also been recently introduced (in their greatly improved condition) into our county, and are quite as popular as the Berkshire.

"I will here give the result of my experience with the Chesters and Berkshires : I procured from a noted breeder in a neighboring State, two Berkshire pigs about ten weeks old, and with them, in a pen, I put two Chester Whites, from a litter of our own, after several of the larger ones had been sold. They were a few days younger than the Berkshires, which were masters at the trough, and they remained so, knocking the Chesters about as though the whites had no rights the blacks were bound to respect. After feeding the four together for seven or eight months, by which time the Chesters weighed seventy-five pounds, each, heavier than the Berkshires, we killed and salted them for our own use, intending to find out which made the best bacon, and we found the Berkshire hams gave more lean meat, though somewhat dry and hard, while that from the Chesters appeared to be more soft and juicy, and was considered much the best for our own eating ; but those who do not like the fat, juicy ham, would prefer the Berkshire, which is also nice.

"It might seem that enough had been written and published in our agricultural papers about the pure bred hogs, when we evidently have no such, and the further we have got from the old English and China type, the better the hog. The Chester White, made in Chester county, Penn.; the Poland-China, made in Butler county, Ohio, lay no claim to any infusion of foreign blood, and are two of the best breeds of hogs in the United States. The black hog, with white feet and a white strip in its face, now called the Berkshire, and the white hog, with thin, curled hair, short head and very crooked face, called Yorkshires, are both very well made and good hogs. The Chester White breed is now the longest established, unmixed with foreign crosses, of any breed with which I am acquainted, and therefore comes nearest a pure bred hog at the present time.

"Some object to them, as being too large for the pork-packers: this I cannot look upon as an objection, as the Chesters will fatten readily at any age, and can furnish any weights the packers may desire (from 200 to 300 lbs.)

"I think they would be more profitable than any small breed, which has to be kept over winter to attain the desired weight, as Chesters, pigged in the spring, will readily attain the desired weights by killing-time in the following fall or winter, and by keeping them longer they can be grown to weigh 600, 800, or even 1,000 pounds. A Chester White exhibited at the Exposition in Philadelphia was said to weigh upwards of 1,300 lbs. live weight.

"We seldom have fatal diseases among our hogs; many of the diseases of swine, as of the sheep, enumerated by the English, I think never occur in this country. As to the Chester Whites being exempt from the attacks of 'cholera,' Thomas Miner, of Edinburgh, Indiana, stated to me some years ago that all his hogs, seventy in number, were attacked with cholera, and the only pig in the whole herd that recovered was a Chester sow, the only one he had. I do not recollect ever hearing of a Chester dying with the cholera, yet I see no reason why they should be exempt. I think we have never had any hog cholera in eastern Pennsylvania, except in a few instances, where pigs were shipped from the West for sale to our dairies."

We have said that the Essex were essentially the same kind of hogs as the Suffolks, except in color and the quality of their skins : The best of the Chester Whites stand in about the same relation to the Poland-Chinas, for if a Chester was partially black, he would easily be mistaken for a Poland-China, and a strictly white Poland-China could scarcely be distinguished from a Chester White.

With many persons who suppose they have had the Chesters in their best estate, there is much prejudice against the breed, but, in many cases, we think the Chesters receive the harshest criticisms from parties who never owned one purely bred, and, in all probability, do not know what they are, or how they should look. Where the best specimens have been handled with the same care, and the same judgment used in mating, breeding, and feeding, that is bestowed on other well-bred, well-fed animals, they have been reasonably satisfactory, and have justly earnest advocates and admirers.

The occasion of the bitterness toward so many hogs that have been called Chester Whites, is that their popularity, and the consequent demand increased, while they were comparatively few in numbers, faster than the supply, which stimulated many unprincipled parties in eastern Pennsylvania to engage in advertising and shipping any white pigs they could obtain, regardless of their character or breeding, and thousands of innocent purchasers of these mongrel pigs supposed they had pure Chesters, and the subsequent failures with them caused no little loss, mortification, and deep-seated disgust with the very name. One firm alone, that perhaps raised some of their pigs, publicly proclaimed that they had shipped annually, for three or four years prior to 1870, from 2,500 to 2,900 pigs, and the advertisements of all such parties intimated, indirectly, that their ability to fill orders for choice selected pigs was unlimited.

A gentleman residing in Chester county, gave the New York Farmers' Club some correct ideas as to the way the business was conducted, as follows :

"I live in Chester county, and know something of the operators in this famous breed of pigs; know something of their business, its extent, and their ability to meet the demand with pure Chester Whites—pigs pure enough to reproduce themselves. There are, no doubt, a great many breeders who keep the stock unmixed, but if you knew the enormous demand from abroad, independent of the local wants, you would see how little likelihood there is of meeting it with pure stock. The consequence is, every nook and corner is scoured for pigs—pigs that are not black, that is all that is required.

"Drovers, hucksters, and almost every other itinerant, are on the lookout for pigs, until they have tripled in price from what they were a few years ago.

"Last fall, a neighbor had several litters of very ordinary pigs, which a farmer engaged at a very young age, to make sure of them; but a hog-dealer—as they are called—came around in a few days, bid higher, and took the most of the lot.

"Another neighbor procured a pair of pigs from one of the breeders we have in the county, and the first litter he raised from them were nearly all more or less spotted with black, thus showing unmistakably bad blood."

When the reaction following this set in, it was, of course, severe. The graceless scamps who followed this business, have given the Chester Whites a much worse reputation than they deserve, and the question as to whether the true Chester White is an established breed, is not worth discussing with those who really know them.

They are appropriately classed with the large breeds, growing, if kept, to almost any size, and hold their white color perfectly under all circumstances. Docility and cleanliness are marked characteristics with them, and the sows make an excellent foundation upon which to cross boars of any of the more refined breeds, the offspring inheriting size from the sow, and early maturity and fine feeding quality from the boar.

The tendency of late years has been to reduce the Chester's coarseness of bone, head, ears and hair; and it is a marked improvement.* Breeders in Ohio and elsewhere have claimed to make variations in the types reared by them during several generations of the stock, entitling it to designation and registry in a separate record as "Improved" Chester Whites, but whether the "improvement" over the best of the Chester county stock, as bred from 1865 to 1880, is a material one, is an open question.

Taking the specimens of the breed shown at the Columbian Exposition in 1893 as representing its best, there was little to indicate that the Chester Whites, at that time, were any improvement on their ancestry of twenty-five years before, and the contrast they presented, alongside many of other breeds, could scarcely impress the unbiased observer as strikingly favorable.

Where farmers have large Chester sows that are too coarse, a cross with a good Suffolk boar will give pigs with fine points and most excellent feeding qualities, fattening readily from the time they are weaned.

We have had considerable experience with the Chesters, perhaps as good as Chester county afforded, and their merits are many, but they were discarded, with other white breeds, for their one failing in the Western climate and under Western treatment, viz., liability to skin diseases, especially *mange.* Harsh treatment and exposure tell severely against the hardiest white hogs, but we believe judicious management and breeding will yet do much to rid them of this apparent tenderness.

---

*The heavy lopped ears, coarse heads, long, coarse tails and hair are much less characteristic of the breed now than they were in its earlier days, while their coats are of silvery white hair of reasonable fineness.

The National Convention adopted the following as their description of the

CHARACTERISTICS AND MARKINGS OF CHESTER WHITES.

"Head short, broad between the eyes; ears thin, projecting forward and lap at the point; neck short and thick; jowl large; body lengthy and deep, broad on back; hams full and deep; legs short, and well set under for bearing the weight; coating thinnish white, straight, and if a little wavy not objectionable; small tail, and no bristles."

CHAPTER V.

THE BERKSHIRES.

For ten years subsequent to 1831 there raged in the United States what might appropriately be called "the Berkshire fever," and mainly from the efforts of those interested in their importation, and sale at fancy prices, the breed became notorious, if not popular. Many substantial farmers, and others, invested in them largely, and no small efforts were made to sustain the mushroom reputation that speculators had made for them, but while they were, even at that time, hogs of excellent breeding and truly valuable, the careless, neglectful systems then in vogue with too many farmers, were not adapted to maintaining the good qualities given the breed by English breeding and feeding, and deterioration followed. Failing to realize the expectations of those who purchased them, a reaction set in, and breeders became disgusted with, and so prejudiced against, the stock and its very name, that they would afterwards scarcely accept of a Berkshire as a present.

Much of the prejudice then engendered only ceased

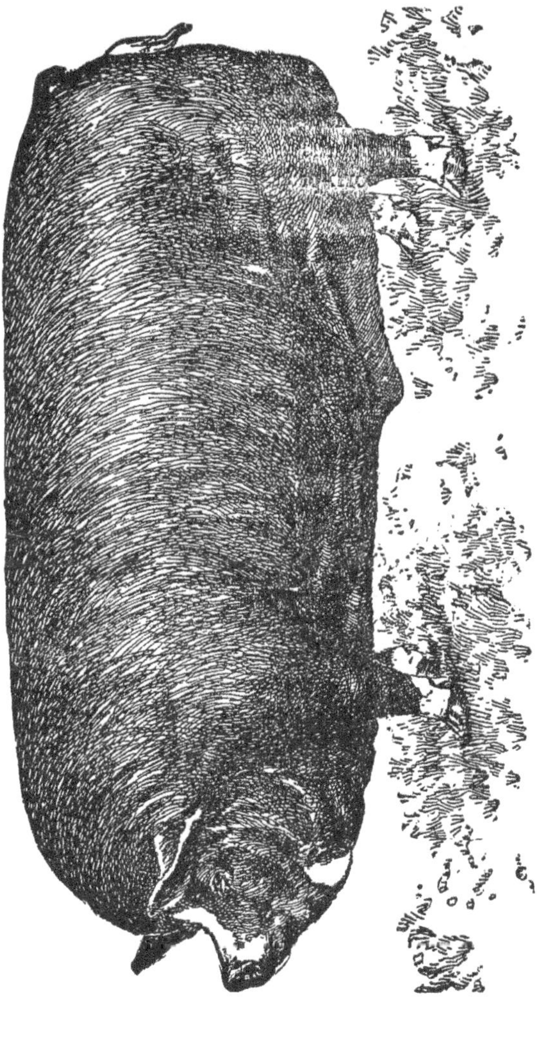

Fig. 3. COLUMBUS, THE GREAT BERKSHIRE SIRE.

with its generation, and perhaps but little or none of it exists at the present time.

Since about 1865, new importations, of the finest specimens of the improved Berkshires that Great Britain could produce, have been made, and the stock has been widely disseminated; being now thoroughly known and appreciated, it probably stands second to none in the estimation of intelligent pork-producers throughout the United States and Canadas.

While the Berkshires of the present time are probably much improved over those of forty years ago, the spirit of improvement is still abroad, and the standard of perfection is placed high.

Prominent among the good qualities that serve to make them favorites are:

1*st.*—Great muscular power and vitality, which render them less liable to disease than many other breeds.

2*d.*—Activity, combined with strong digestive and assimilating powers; hence they return a maximum amount of flesh and fat for the food consumed.

3*d.*—The sows are unequalled for prolificacy, and as careful nurses and good sucklers.

4*th.*—The pigs are strong, smart, and active at birth, and consequently less liable to mishaps.

5*th.*—They can be fattened for market at any time, while they may be fed to any reasonable weight desired.

6*th.*—Their flesh is the highest quality of pork.

7*th.*—Power of the boar to transmit the valuable qualities of the breed to its progeny, when used as a cross.

8*th.*—Their unsurpassed uniformity in color, marking, and quality.

It is doubtful if any hogs are nearer thoroughbred, in its best sense, or more certain to reproduce themselves with fidelity than the improved Berkshires. Crossed with Poland-Chinas they make *the best feeding hogs possible*—in fact, there is scarcely a medium or large breed upon which they cannot be crossed with advantage, owing to their great vigor and hardiness.

In our own breeding and feeding operations, no breed has been found so eminently satisfactory as the best Berkshires, and we breed them pure in considerable numbers for feeding purposes, having years ago discontinued the raising of any others.

Their reasonable size, quick growth, easy fattening, docility, uniformity, and hardiness captivated us, and every day's experience but adds to our admiration of them.

The pigs, even when coming in the most unfavorable seasons, have a tenacity of hold on life that is truly wonderful.

Many of the meanest hogs and those of the worst disposition that we have known were *called* Berkshires, but they sustained about the same relation to the true sort, that the propagators of them did to intelligent farmers and breeders.

The Berkshires having become so numerous, and their excellence so generally recognized, the friends of the breed organized in March, 1875, at Springfield, Illinois, the "American Berkshire Association," having for its object the "collection, preservation, and dissemination of reliable information on the origin, breeding, and management of Berkshire swine, and the publication of a Herd Book, or Record of Berkshire pedigrees."

One of the first steps of the Association was to offer a premium of $100 for the best approved orignal essay on the origin and management of Berkshires. The premium was awarded to A. B. Allen, Esq., of New York, the historical and descriptive portions of whose essay are presented in subsequent pages.

The entire essay appears in Vol. I of the "American Berkshire Record," and we are safe in saying that the subject has not, in any other published paper, been treated by any one so thoroughly familiar with it as Mr.

Allen, and we give a considerable portion of it here in lieu of any attempt to treat the subject ourselves.

Mr. Allen prepared the report on Berkshires, as adopted by the "Swine Breeders' Convention;" but we omit it, as the essay contains the same, and considerable other information.

The Convention agreed upon the following as the

CHARACTERISTICS AND MARKINGS OF BERKSHIRES.

Color black, with white on feet, face, tip of tail, and an occasional splash of white on the arm; while a small spot of white on some other part of the body does not argue an impurity of blood, yet it is to be discouraged to the end that uniformity of color may be attained by breeders; white upon one ear, or a bronze or copper spot on some part of the body argues no impurity, but rather a reappearance of original colors. Markings of white other than those named above are suspicious, and a pig so marked should be rejected.

Face short, fine, and well dished, broad between the eyes; ears generally almost erect, but sometimes inclining forward with advancing age, small, thin, soft, and showing veins; jowl full; neck short and thick; shoulder short from neck, to middling deep from back down; back broad and straight, or a very little arched; ribs—long ribs, well sprung, giving rotundity of body; short ribs of good length, giving breadth and levelness of loins; hips good length from point of hip to rump; hams thick, round, and deep, holding their thickness well back and down to the hocks; tail fine and small, set on high up; legs short and fine, but straight and very strong, with hoofs erect, legs set wide apart; size medium; length medium, extremes are to be avoided; bone fine and compact; offal very light; hair fine and compact; skin pliable.

The Berkshires are hardy, prolific, and excellent nurses;

their meat is of superior quality, with fat and lean well mixed.

As showing the weight that animals of this breed will attain at an early age, it is stated that J. A. Brown, of Milton, Illinois, sold, in 1873, a lot of Berkshire pigs of an average age of nine months, and their average weight was 305 pounds.

As indicating the estimate placed on this breed in England, the leading work of that country on swine raising says :*

"Among the black breeds, by universal consent, the improved Berkshire hog stands at the head of the list, either to breed pure, or to cross with inferior breeds. * * * They are now considered, by Berkshire farmers, to be divided into a middle (medium size) and a small breed. If first-class, they should be well covered with long, black, silky hair. * * * The white should be confined to four white feet, a white spot between the eyes, and a few white hairs behind each shoulder."

PREMIUM ESSAY.

BY A. B ALLEN.

THE ORIGINAL BREED OF BERKSHIRE SWINE

"Tradition, and the earliest published accounts of what has long been particularly distinguished by the name of Berkshire swine, represents them, down to about a century since, as among the largest breeds of England, weighing, full grown, from 700 to 1,000 pounds, or more. The 'Complete Grazier' describes one, in 1807, as weighing 113 stone, (904 lbs.) This was exhibited, with others, by Sir William Curtis, at the cattle show of Lord Somerville, in that year. Johnson, in his 'Farmers' Encyclopædia,' London, 1842, says that they weighed at that time from 50 to 100 stone (400 to 800 lbs. The latter of these, doubtless, were of the improved breed.

"Originally, they were represented as being generally of a buff, sandy, or reddish-brown color, spotted with black, occasionally tawny or white spotted in the same manner. They were coarse in the bone; head rather large, with heavy flop ears; broad on the

* Sidney's "Youatt on the Pig," London, 1860.

back; deep in the chest; flat-sided, and long in the body; thick and heavy in both shoulders and hams; well let down in the twist; bristles and long curly hair, with rather short, strong legs. Their meat was better marbled than that of any other breed of swine in Great Britain—that is, had a greater proportion of lean freely intermixed with fine streaks of fat, which makes it much more tender and juicy than it would otherwise be. They were consequently, from time immemorial, preferred to all other swine there, for choice hams, shoulders, and bacon. They were slow feeders, and did not ordinarily mature till two and a half to three years old.

"It is thus that I find the Berkshire hog figured and described in the earliest English publications to which I have been able, thus far, to obtain access. But in the second volume of the magnificent folio edition, illustrated with colored plates, now lying before me, of 'The Breeds of the Domestic Animals of the British Islands,' by Professor David Low, published in London, in 1842, is a portrait of a Berkshire as I have described above, except being of rounder body and somewhat finer in all his points, with ears like most of those of modern breeding, medium in size, and erect, instead of flopping. This portrait is of a sandy or reddish-brown color, spotted with black; the feet and legs for nearly their whole length, white, slightly streaked on the sides and behind, with reddish-brown. It, of course, represents one of the old breed considerably improved, and marked as I occasionally found them in all my visits to Berkshire down to 1867. But the pigs which I saw thus marked were of the same size and shape, and as fine in all their points, as a general run of the black, slate, or plum colors of the present day.

"FORMATION OF THE IMPROVED BERKSHIRE SWINE.

"Tradition tells us that this was made by a cross of the black, or deep plum-colored Siamese boar, on the old unimproved Berkshire sows. Other traditions assert that the black and white spotted, and even pure white Chinese boar was also sparingly used to assist in the same purpose. I can well believe this; for I often saw swine in Berkshire spotted, about half and half black and white, in addition to the reddish-brown, or buff and black, and so on almost up to the pure plum color or black. The produce of the above cross or crosses was next bred together, and by judicious subsequent selections, the improved breed, as we now find it, became, in due time, fixed and permanent in all its desirable points.

"Another feature, aside from the half and half black and white spots hitherto occasionally found to mark the improved Berkshire swine, which may be adduced in support of the supposition of a sparing cross with the white and light spotted Chinese, is the shape of the jowls. All these which I have bred in my piggery, or imported at different times direct from China, or have seen elsewhere, had much fuller and fatter jowls than the Siamese. Some of the breeders of England preferred the fat jowls, because carrying the most meat; others the leaner, as they said this gave their stock a finer and higher bred look in the head.

"THE SIAMESE SWINE.

"In the same volume of Professor Low, which contains the Berkshire portrait as described above, is a colored plate of a Siamese sow. She is a dark-slate, varying to that of a rich plum color. The two hind feet are white; the fore legs and feet white, shaded in front with plum. The face is dished; head fine, with short erect ears; shoulders and hams extra large; back broad, with a deep, round, and longish body. The sow is represented with a slightly swayed or hollow back, at which we need not wonder, considering its length, and that she has a litter of nine great fat pigs tugging away at her dugs. These, Professor Low says, were got by a half-bred Chinese boar, which, I presume, from the color of the pigs, was white; for some of them were pure white, while others are mixed with slate, or plum and white, and one is a buff, with black spots, like the original Berkshire.

"I will now describe the Siamese swine, such as I possessed and bred for several years on my farm. They varied in color from deep rich plum to dark-slate and black; had two to three white feet, but no white on the legs or other parts of the body. The head was short and fine, with a dished face, and rather thin jowls; ears short, slender, and erect; shoulders and hams round, smooth, and extra large; back broad and somewhat arched, except in sows heavy with pig or suckling pigs, but even then it was straight rather than swayed; body of moderate length, deep, well ribbed up, and nearly as round as a barrel; chest deep and broad; twist well let down; legs fine and short; tail very slender and well set, with a handsome curl in it near the rump; hair soft, silky, and thin; no bristles even on the boars; skin thin and of a dark hue, yet when scalded, scraped white; flesh firm, sweet, and very tender, with less lean than in the Berkshire. Although so compact, round and smooth in build, they had a fine, high-bred, up-headed style, especially in their walk, which instantly attracted the attention of all who called to see them. They were moderately prolific, and as hardy as any other breed of swine I ever kept, the extremes of heat and cold never injuring them. They were gentle in disposition, very quiet, and easily kept, and would partially fatten on good pasture, or coarse, raw vegetables. They could be made fit for the butcher at any age; matured at 12 to 15 months old; and when fully fattened, generally weighed from 250 to 300 pounds, occasionally going to 350, or 400 pounds. They had very fine bones and light offal.

"It was, doubtless, with Siamese boars as perfect as I have described, that the cross was made on the original Berkshire sows, which has contributed so largely to the formation of the improved breed, held in such high estimation for a full century or more past.

"WHEN WAS THE CROSS FIRST MADE?

"Several aged men in different parts of Berkshire, of whom I inquired on my first visit to England, in 1841, informed me that they had known there improved swine of the same type as I then found them, from earliest childhood. But the most particular, and apparently reliable, account I was able to obtain, was from Mr. Westbrook, of Pinckney Green, Bysham, who told me that his father possessed them as early as the year 1780, in as great perfection as the best then existing in the country. Thus it will be seen that the improvement is now at least a century old, and more probably a century and a quarter; for it would have taken some years back of 1780 to begin a new breed of swine, and get it up to a fixed type at that period.

"CHARACTERISTICS OF THE BEST OF THE IMPROVED BERKSHIRE SWINE AT THIS TIME.

"Snout and head fine and rather short, but larger in proportion to the body in the male than in the female, and with a bolder and more determined expression; face dished and broad between the eyes; jowls full or thinner, according to the fancy of the breeder; eyes bright and expressive; ears small, thin, and upright, or inclining their points a little forward; neck short, rather full in the throat, and harmoniously swelling to the shoulders; chest broad and deep; back broad and moderately arched; rump nearly level with it; well let down in the twist: body of good length and depth, round, with well sprung ribs, and straight along the sides and under the belly; shoulders, above all, in the boar, extra thick, yet sloping smoothly to the body; hams broad, round, deep, and so thick through from side to side, particularly in the sow and barrow, that, standing directly behind, except when pretty fat, the sides of the body are scarcely seen between them and the shoulders; legs fine, strong, of moderate length, and set rather wide apart; feet small, with clear, tough hoofs; tail slender and well set, with a handsome curl near the rump; bones fine and of an ivory-like grain and hardness; offal very light in comparison to weight of carcass; hair fine, soft, and silky; no bristles, even on the boar; skin thin and mellow, with elastic handling of the flesh beneath; quick and spirited in movement; stylish in carriage, and, in the boar, more especially, bold and imposing in presence.

"COLOR AND MARKING.

"The most favorite color among the best breeders in Berkshire, in 1841, was a deep rich plum, with a slight flecking on the body of white, or a little mingling with it of buff; a small blaze in the face; two to four feet white, and more or less white hair in the tail. The plum color was preferred to the black or slate, because it carried rather higher style and finer points with it, a superior quality of flesh, softer hair, and thinner skin.

"The above is no ideal description of choice improved Berkshire swine, for I found several such in traversing the country, and purchased and sent them home, to grace my own piggery. Nor, with all these points, were they lacking in size; and to substantiate this assertion, I will here note the dimensions of one of those I imported at this time, which I called 'Windsor Castle,' he having been bred and reared near that magnificent royal residence, standing in Berkshire.

"As he lay down he measured, in a direct line along the side, from the tip of his nose to the end of his rump, six feet three and a half inches. If measured standing up, with his head stooping towards the ground, by running the tape line from the tip of his nose over the head between the ears, and along the back to the end of the rump, as swine are often measured, it would have made upwards of seven feet long; but I do not consider this a fair way of measuring. Hight to top of the shoulder, two feet eleven inches; hight to top of rump, three feet; girth close behind the shoulders, five feet six inches. He was in rather lean condition when I measured him, as I kept him so in order not to be too heavy to serve small sows. It is well known that when a Berkshire is fully fed, in addition to the meat on his sides, he lays two to four inches more on his back. I am confident if 'Windsor Castle' had been altered to a barrow, and fully fattened, he would then have measured three feet and two inches high to top of shoulder, and three feet three inches high to top of rump; would have girthed around the heart seven feet, and weighed, dressed, at least eight hundred pounds. He was as fine in hair and all his points, and as good a handler as the choicest of those of smaller size; and for a combination of size, style, vigor, and noble presence, he exceeded anything I ever saw or ever expect to see in the *genus Sus.* A friend of mine, who was a special nice judge and breeder of horses and cattle, but who hated hogs, and would go as far to kick one as the celebrated late John Randolph, of Roanoke, Virginia, was in the habit of declaring he would go to kick a sheep; on visiting my piggery and seeing 'Windsor Castle,' was so surprised and delighted with his superb appearance, that he exclaimed he was the only one of this sort of stock he had ever looked upon which had any *poetry* in him, and that for his sake alone he should henceforth be reconciled to swine.

"SIZE OF THE IMPROVED BERKSHIRE.

"I have heard of those, both in England and America, whose dead weight, dressed, occasionally exceeded 800 lbs.; but at the time I first visited the former country, the general weight, full grown, was about the same as at the present time—namely, from 300 to 600 lbs.; according as the smaller or larger pigs were selected from the litters for fattening, and as they were subsequently fed and attended. The smaller sizes matured several months the quickest, and were preferred in the markets for fresh pork; and for curing also, for those who were particularly nice in the choice of their meat, being rather more tender and delicate than the larger animals.

"QUALITY OF MEAT.

"The meat of the improved Berkshire, like that of the unimproved, abounds in a much greater proportion of sweet, tender, juicy lean, well marbled with very fine streaks of fat, than other breeds of swine; but the former is far more delicate now, than the latter ever was. This renders the whole carcass the most suitable of all for smoking. The hams and shoulders are almost entirely lean, a thin rim of fat covering only the outside.

"MATURITY.

"The improved Berkshire could be fattened at any age. Barrows matured in 12 to 18 months, according as selected from the litters, whether the largest or smallest, and as subsequently fed and treated. It took boars and sows reserved for breeding about six months longer to get their fullest size and weight, not being pushed by high feed so rapidly as those destined for more immediate slaughter.

"EARLIEST IMPORTATIONS INTO AMERICA.

"The first importation into the country, of which I find record, was made in 1823, by Mr. John Brentnall, an English farmer who settled in English Neighborhood, New Jersey. I became acquainted with his sons after their removal to Orange county, New York, and purchased of them stock descended from this importation.

"The next were imported in 1832, by Mr. Siday Hawes, an English farmer who settled in Albany, New York. He subsequently made other importations, some of the descendants of all which I added to the stock on my farm.

"I have heard that by the year 1838, a few followed into Canada and some of the Western States, from England. I bought a small lot that came into western New York in 1839; and late that year, Messrs. Bagg & Wait, English farmers who had settled in Orange county, New York, began their large importation, which they continued for several years, disposing of them mainly in Kentucky, Tennessee, Missouri, and the South. In 1841 I selected in Berkshire, England, and imported into New York, upwards of forty head of the choicest of the Improved Breed of swine I could find there. The above have been followed by numerous other importations down to the present time, both into the United States and Canada. Those curious as to the particulars of these will find them pretty fully recorded in the various Agricultural journals of America. * * * *

"ADVANTAGE IN MAINTAINING THE BERKSHIRE BREED.

"There is a growing taste on the part of the American people, coinciding with that which has been cultivated a long time in Europe, for tender, juicy, well marbled, smoked hams, shoulders, and side pieces, in preference to very fat, salt pork. This should be encouraged, as the former are not only the more palatable to persons in general, but are unquestionably the most healthy food. Considering these facts, the Berkshire, above all others, should be the favorite swine among us; and we ought to take all possible pains in breeding, rearing, and fattening them in such a manner as to make a superior quality of smoked meat, not only for the home, but also for the foreign market.

"Improved methods of curing and packing should likewise be adopted, so as to enable us to get as high a price in the English market as the best Irish bacon commands. This, I find often quoted 20 to 30 per cent above American.

"Indian corn, which in the United States grows in such abundance, is undoubtedly superior to anything which can be produced in Ireland, for making the best quality of *fat pork;* but I have heard this questioned as to *hams* and *bacon.* Some feeders contend that fine, mealy potatoes, cooked and mixed with barley, oats, peas, or beans, or several of these, fed together, will produce a superior quality of bacon. This is a matter worth inquiring into, and I would suggest an earnest consideration of it on the part of our feeders, and of those engaged also in bacon curing and packing. The Irish have one advantage over the Americans, in the English market; and that is in being so much nearer to it, they can cure their bacon and offer it on sale in a fresher and milder state than we are able to at present. If we should, on trial, hereafter find that it can be sent forward at a profit, in refrigerators, kept down to a low and even temperature, we could then probably obtain as high prices in the English market as do the Irish, and thus add another desirable item to the exports of America."

CHAPTER VI.

THE SUFFOLKS.

The Suffolks are not raised pure, or used as a cross in the principal pork producing States so extensively as several other breeds, nor are they so well known to a majority of farmers, who have a belief, if not positive knowledge, that they are somewhat delicate, and difficult to raise.

The objections to them are, that they are not large enough, not satisfactory as breeders and nurses, and that their skins are too tender, and thinly haired, to withstand the exposure to which the average farmer's hogs are subjected.

As to size, the best strains of Suffolks are large enough for those who prefer to raise hogs of medium weights, while for quietness, and easy keeping qualities, no breed

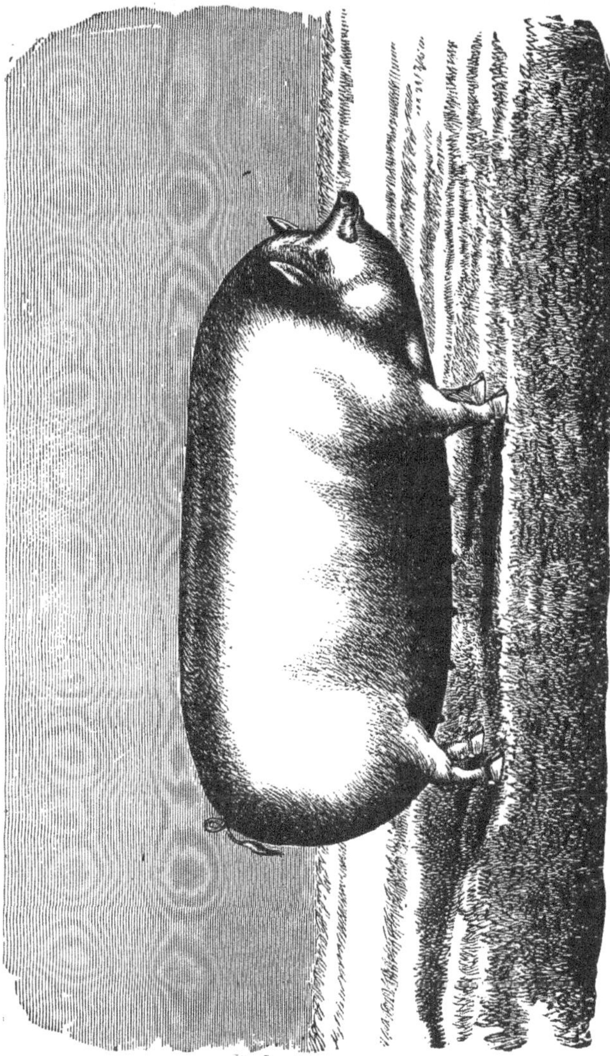

Fig. 4.—SUFFOLK SOW.

of swine can excel them, and to those who like *pets*, we would recommend a cleanly-kept Suffolk pig in preference to any "poodle," or other diminutive canine, we ever saw. The sows are not so prolific, so regular as breeders, nor usually so good sucklers as others that mature less early, and not so predisposed to excessive fatness while young.

Experience with the Suffolks has convinced many that the wind, sun, and mud, make sad work with their tender, papery skins, and we have seen them, when reasonably well kept, become chapped and cracked all over, and the smaller pigs so mangy and sore as to present the appearance of a solid scab. Of course, all Suffolks are not so affected, and we think that in many localities, they are no more liable to suffer in this way than hogs of any other white breed. The climate of some Western and Southwestern States is unmistakably severe on white hogs, not well haired, and when such are constantly exposed to biting frosts, drying winds, and scorching sun, the results will, in most cases, be anything but satisfactory, and the balance will be found on the wrong side of the ledger.

As now bred, we cannot look upon them as a reasonably profitable hog for general use, but Suffolk boars can be used to good advantage on many farms where white hogs are preferred, and more refinement is desired.

The Hon. John Wentworth, of Cook county, Illinois, having bred the Suffolks, exclusively, for upwards of twenty years, owning many of the finest in the world, and being, after this long experience, an enthusiastic admirer of them, we solicited his estimate of them as a farmer's hog, and he gives the following in reply:

"After trying carefully all the other breeds, we give the preference to the Suffolks, and we think all others will who try them as long and as impartially as we have. They make the most pork with the least food, and with the least bone. They are the quietest hogs. Give them enough to eat and they will never leave the premises. They lie down and remain so until they want more food. They make the least offal of any hogs, and they root about the least, even when short of food. For crossing upon other hogs, they have decidedly the preference. Their cross upon the largest white sows make the best of Chester Whites. Their crosses upon the largest black, or speckled sows, make the equals of Berkshires, Magies, Polands, Poland-Chinas, Essex, Byfield, and other dark-colored breeds.

"Indeed, with a judicious crossing of the Suffolk boar upon the ordinary cheap hogs of the country, you can closely imitate any existing breed of hogs, or make a breed of any form you please.

"It is a remarkable fact that the Chesters, Berkshires, Magies, Polands, Poland-Chinas, Essex, Byfields, etc., etc., as well as the later formed breeds that have taken the most prizes, have been manufactured in this way, from the Suffolks, which are the oldest breed known to man. Our Suffolks are well haired, and run in our pastures and barn-yards with our cattle, sheep, geese, ducks, and chickens. They are as quiet and harmless as any animals we keep. As the Suffolk is not a new breed, nor recently made up from unknown crosses, but a long-established English variety, it is therefore a true breeder. In them there is no breeding back to the original common or made-up stock. Their litters are not part of one kind and part of another, but they are uniformly true to the Suffolk characteristics. They breed even, each pig as good as another. * * * * * During the season of grass they will keep fat without any other food. Suffolk pork costs less and brings more money than any other.

"Suffolks are the most popular breed in England. The Suffolk attains maturity at an early age, and may always be in a condition to kill from the time they are a month old. The carcasses command a considerable extra price over the common hogs of the country, partly on account of the greater weight in proportion to the bone, and partly from the pork being of better quality and flavor. It derives its well-known name, "the English nobleman's hog," from the fact that it is always in a condition to be killed, however suddenly company comes.

"The object of the farmer is to get the most meat to the least bone, the most valuable matter in the hog upon the same food to the least portion of the valueless matter. The Suffolk may be small, compared with mammoth breeds, but he contains as much that is eatable as most hogs of double his weight, and which consume four times his food. But the Suffolk can be made of superior size by keeping off its flesh until the bones are properly developed, and this development cannot take place whilst the young bones are overladen with flesh, as those of over-fatted Suffolks are apt to be. But, owing to their short legs, they weigh much more than is generally supposed. The Suffolks never root up their pastures, nor make enemies of neighbors by wandering away from home, or by breaking into their premises. The Suffolks are invariably white, except now and then one will have two or three bluish spots. These bluish spots, on the skin, but never in the hair, unlike those found upon any other hogs, indicate purity of blood and recent importation.

"We started out in 1855 with Suffolks descended from the pens of Lord Wenlock and Mr. Crisp, of England; and we can safely say that we have bred from every importation into the United States and the Provinces since; and we intend to keep up our stock by importing ourselves and availing ourselves of the importations of others. We have sold Suffolks into every State and Territory, the Empire of Japan, the Sandwich Islands, the British Provinces, and Mexico.

"The following statement will explain how persons who annually ship large quantities of hogs to Chicago view the characteristics of the Suffolk. When we first began to breed Suffolks, and there were no railroads in the country, hog raisers would only buy boars and raise half-breeds to drive. As railroads approached them they would raise three-quarters blooded to drive. As railroads would reach them, and they had little or no distance to drive, they have bought Suffolk sows as well as boars, and raised full-bloods."

Mr. Wentworth, in a communication to the "*Prairie Farmer*," says:

"I read, with great interest, the report of the committee at the late Swine Breeders' Association upon the characteristics of the Suffolk hogs. I have had them exclusively for the past eighteen years, and my sales will average one hundred every year for the past ten years, and I think I have had all the importations represented in my herd.

"While I commend the general correctness of the report, I would state that there is one characteristic that was not only not alluded to by the committee, but it was rather repudiated in the following words, 'free from spots or any other color.' Now there is a liability in all Suffolks to have round bluish spots upon their skins, although covered with white bristles, and these spots seem to increase with age. My present boar was selected for me by Mr. Harison, Secretary of the New York State Agricultural Society. When he arrived, aged about six months, he was spot less, and so continued until about two years of age, and then bluish spots of the size of an old-fashioned silver dollar commenced growing upon him. Now, at four years of age, he has about twenty of them, although the bristles covering them are white. Of course, these spots are exceptions, not one in ten having them, and very few inside of one year old; yet there is a tendency to them and no hog should be rejected as a pure Suffolk on their account. These spots are easily detected from black spots.

"At one of the State Fairs at Chicago, one of my boars not only took the first premium as the best Suffolk, but the sweepstake prize as the best boar of any age or breed upon the ground. He had several of these spots upon him at that time, although having none until he was a year old. I notice these bluish spots occasionally upon hogs at the stock yards, which have, in all respects, characteristics of the Suffolks.

"A correspondent of yours, whilst finding fault with the size of the Suffolk, thinks they are the best for crossing upon other hogs. I have found this to be the invariable opinion of men who want a breed of hogs of their own, independent of everybody else. Wherever they start, whatever may be their groundwork, before they get through making their new breed of hogs they invariably incorporate somewhere a cross of the Suffolk.

"Your paper says that four hundred is the profitable size of the hog. The Suffolks can easily be made to weigh this amount, by feeding them lightly until their legs have acquired sufficient strength to support their weight of carcass. The inferior weight attributed so often to Suffolks arises entirely from overfeeding them when young."

Mr. William Smith, of Detroit, Michigan, has long occupied a front rank as a breeder of these hogs, and is familiar with them and their breeding, in England, as well as America, and his testimony is this:

"Having bred the Suffolks continually for over forty years, I can safely assert that they are a great favorite with me. I find in the improved breed nothing to condemn, and everything to commend. They attain good size at an early age, and their quiet, pleasant disposition, clean, snow-white appearance, and handsome form, are very desirable features in connection with their many other good qualities, not the least of which is the comparative small amount of food they require.

"The Suffolks are rapidly gaining in favor, and wherever introduced give good satisfaction. They are quite hardy and thrive in almost any climate that any of their species will, from the most northern part of Canada to southern Missouri and California. We know that they flourish and give satisfaction, as hundreds of my customers can testify.

"Canada, Michigan, New York, parts of Ohio, Indiana, Illinois, Iowa, and other States, are rapidly becoming stocked with them, and in my opinion it will not be many years before they become "the hog" of the country. There is no possible question about their being *the very best thoroughbred* for improving the common or native breeds, and for this quality alone they would be entitled to a front rank in the list of valuable breeds."

The Report adopted by the "National Convention of Swine Breeders" on Suffolk swine, is as follows:

"Mr. Sidney says: Yorkshire stands in the first rank as a pig breeding county, possessing the largest white breed in England as well as an excellent medium and small breed, all white, the last of which, transplanted into the south, has figured and won prizes under the names of divers noblemen and gentlemen, and in more than one county. The Yorkshires are closely allied with the Cumberland breeds, and have been so much intermixed that, with the exception of the very largest breeds, it is difficult to tell where the Cumberland begins and where the Yorkshire ends. It will be enough to say, for the present, that the modern Manchester boar, the improved Suffolk, the improved Middlesex, the Coleshill, and the Prince Albert or Windsor, were all founded on Yorkshire-Cumberland stock, and some of them are merely pure Yorkshires transplanted and re-christened.

Speaking of pigs kept in the dairy district of Cheshire, he says, 'white pigs have not found favor with the dairymen of Cheshire, and the white ones most used are Manchester boars, another name for the Yorkshire-Cumberland breed.' He says, in another place, and all the authors who have followed him, down to the latest published work on the subject, occupy space in describing various county pigs, which have long ceased to possess, if ever they possessed, any merit worthy of the attention of the breeder. Thus the Norfolk, the Suffolk, the Bedford, the Cheshire, have each separate notice, not one of which, except the Suffolk, is worthy of cultivation, and the Suffolk is only another name for a small Yorkshire pig.

"CHARACTERISTICS AND MARKINGS OF SUFFOLKS.

"Head small, very short; cheeks prominent and full; face dished; snout small and very short; jowl fine; ears short, small, thin, upright, soft, and silky; neck very short and thick, the head appearing almost as if set on front of shoulders; no arching of crest; chest wide and deep—elbows standing out; brisket wide but not deep; shoulders thick, rather upright, rounding outwards from top to elbow; crops wide and full; sides and flanks, long ribs, well arched out from back, good length between; shoulders and hams, flank well filled out, and coming well down at ham; back broad, level, and straight from crest to tail, no falling off or down at tail; hams wide and full, well rounded out, twist very wide and full all the way down; legs small and very short, standing wide apart, in sows just keeping belly from the ground; bone fine; feet small, hoofs rather spreading; tail small, long, and tapering; skin thin, of a pinkish shade, free from color; hair fine and silky, not too thick; color of hair pale yellowish white, perfectly free from any spots or other color; size small to medium."

Since about 1882 several gentlemen, particularly in Eastern States, have taken much interest in what are designated as "Small Yorkshires." They are neat little white hogs, with wonderfully short, dished faces, and so much like the Suffolks that some persons who raise both confess they can scarcely distinguish them apart. Their similarity is so great that, as a matter of fact, a Suffolk makes a very good small Yorkshire, and *vice versa.*

CHAPTER VII.

THE ESSEX.

The Essex breed of swine is comparatively unknown among the general farmers of the Mississippi Valley, and we have no knowledge of their being raised in any considerable numbers for pork. Still, in some localities, they are bred in a limited way—more, perhaps, in Kentucky, than elsewhere—and we have never encountered a person who had once tried them, who did not place a high estimate on their value as a small breed, and especially on the boars to use for crossing on sows of larger breeds.

They seem to be essentially the same as the Suffolks, except in their black color, and less liability to skin diseases, which would in a majority of cases make them the favorites over their white competitors.

We think there is small probability that the Essex swine, as now bred, will ever become the prevailing breed, from the fact that they are of a smaller class of hogs than most farmers care to raise, or packers to buy and handle, and we deem it improbable that the next fifty or one hundred years will witness the raising of smaller swine, generally, than the Berkshires, and it is more than likely that, in the future, the happy medium will be an animal in size between the best modeled small-boned Berkshire and the coarser Poland-Chinas of the present time.

Just here, perhaps, is a fitting place to remark—and we do so after full deliberation—that the party who can exhibit at the *next* Centennial Exposition any better feeding hogs, or those better suited for general purposes than a cross between the two last-named breeds, will have some stock to be *very proud of.*

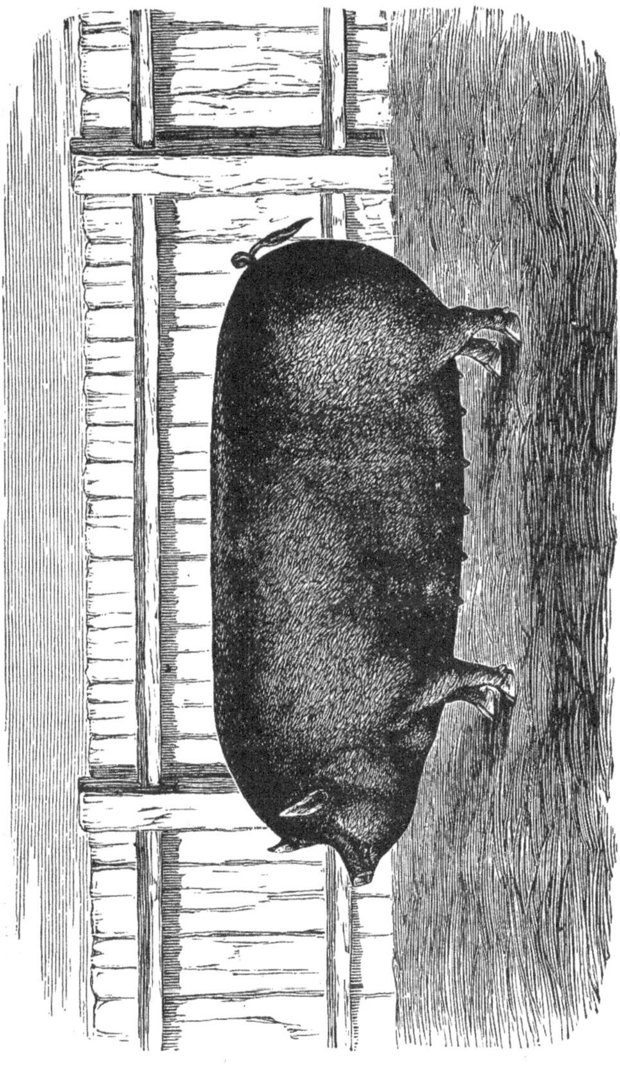

Fig. 5.—ESSEX SOW.

Sidney's "Youatt on the Pig," (London, 1860), says:

"Early maturity, and an excellent quality of flesh, are among the merits of the improved Essex. * * *

"The defect of the improved Essex is a certain delicacy, probably arising from their southern descent, and an excessive aptitude to fatten, which, unless carefully counteracted by exercise and diet, often diminishes the fertility of the sows, and causes difficulty in rearing the young.

"As before observed, they are invaluable as a cross, being sure to give quality and early maturity to any breed, and especially valuable when applied to a black breed, where porkers are required. For this purpose they have been extensively and successfully used, in all the black pig districts of this country, [Great Britain,] where, as well as in France and Germany, and in the United States, they have superseded the use of the imported Neapolitan and Chinese.

"Many attempts, on a limited scale, to perpetuate the breed pure, have been unsatisfactory, because it is too pure to stand in-and-in breeding. They require much care when young.

"In the sows, the paternal fattening properties are apt to overbalance the milking qualities, and make them bad nurses. * * *

"The improved Essex are ranked amongst the small breeds, and there they are most profitable; but exceptional specimens have been exhibited at agricultural shows in the classes for large breeds."

Mr. Wm. Smith (before quoted under Suffolks) breeds the Essex extensively, near Detroit, Mich., and writes of them thus:

"This is a breed that will be appreciated in proportion as it becomes known. Their characteristics are almost identical with those of the Suffolks, except that the Suffolks are a pure white, while the Essex are a beautiful jet black. This is always the case, and any mixture of color, in either, is inadmissible. The style, form, size, disposition, and feeding qualities are similar in the improved breeds; and the pork of the Essex will dress as white as any, if rightly managed. Although they are considered one of the oldest established breeds, yet there have been frequent and marked improvements within the past fifty years,—not the least of which has been reached during the present decade.

"To Lord Western, of Mark's Hall, Essex, England, is given the credit for their first great improvement, or I might say, of being the originator of the present type, though it was much inferior to

know of none that will give better satisfaction than the Essex."

CHARACTERISTICS AND MARKINGS OF ESSEX.

The report adopted by the Convention of Swine Breeders, of characteristics of this breed, is as follows:

"The Essex is a black hog, originating in the south of England. They are of small to medium in size, and are extensively used in England to cross on the large, coarse swine, to improve their fattening qualities.

"The best specimens may be known as follows: Color black; face short and dishing; ears small, soft, and stand erect while young, but coming down somewhat as they get age; carcass long, broad, straight, and deep; ham heavy and well let down; bone fine; carcass, when fat, composed mostly of lard; hair, ordinarily rather thin. The fattening qualities being very superior As breeders they are very prolific, and are fair nurses."

Since the foregoing was prepared, we have received from Mr. E. W. Cottrell, of Greenfield, Mich., the following, under date of December 15th, 1876:

"Yes; I will cheerfully give you my estimate of the Essex, and will premise by saying, that during my experience in breeding and managing thorough-bred pigs for the past ten years, I have, some of the time, exceeded a a thousand choice animals of the improved breeds, including the Essex in considerable numbers, which has given me an opportunity to compare and experiment upon their relative merits, under the same and different treatment, alongside of each other. I also have intimate knowledge of the experience of a gentleman who has bred these pigs, with others, for the past forty years, both in this country and in England.

"As a result of this experience, I can say that, in my estimation, they take rank among the best.

"The Essex are as distinct from all other types as it is

possible for one breed to differ from another, and still possess the principal valuable features belonging to the species. In form, quality, and disposition, they more nearly resemble the Suffolk than any other breed, and, in fact, there is a similarity between them in this respect.

"In the improved breed, the style, form, color, size, disposition, and general characteristics, are very uniform. They are certainly a standard breed, and one of the oldest established. Mr. William Smith, of Detroit, has been the most extensive importer and breeder of them that I know, and they have always been favorites with him, both here and in England, where he has successfully competed with the most noted breeders. His thorough knowledge and experience has enabled him to give the breed a still higher value than they possessed, even before.

"They mature early, their meat is excellent, and a year, at most, should suffice to feed them to the most profitable condition for pork; which is one of their merits, and when fat, the carcass should yield a large proportion of lard.

"They are invariably black; should have a short, dished face; soft, fine, ears when young, though with age they will begin to grow heavier, and droop somewhat. The body should be of medium length, broad, deep and straight; with a heavy ham, well let down, and bone fine, but strong enough to support the carcass in good style. When in condition, the proportions should always be symmetrical and pleasing; medium, well-haired, with a fine and comparatively soft coat.

"They possess powers of transmitting to their progeny an excess of their own good qualities, when crossed upon common and coarser swine, and the first cross upon our natives will improve their qualities, almost beyond recognition. Excepting the Suffolks, there is no breed that can compare with them for this purpose.

"As breeders and nurses, they are very fair, though not equal to the Berkshires. In fact, all thorough-bred animals, as they become refined, or 'high bred,' lessen their fecund propensities to a greater or less extent ; but ordinarily, with good management, no serious difficulty need be experienced on this point with well bred Essex. It is essential, however, that the brood sows be matured, and not permitted to become too fat, which latter is often apt to be the case, with good feed and treatment.

"Good pasture, with plenty of water, will keep them in ample condition for breeding, throughout the whole grazing season. In fact, I have known them to come out of a good clover field in the fall, 'killing fat,' without having had any other feed. They are good graziers, and have the advantage over some of the more tender-skinned white hogs, of being able to withstand, (at any age, however young,) the hottest sun of July or August, without having their backs or skin in the least affected, and they are never known to scald or mange.

"The young pigs of the Essex are usually more delicate than those of the coarser breeds, and will often appear quite inferior to the latter, at the same age, up to eight or ten weeks, when they will begin to shoot ahead, and 'show their breeding.' This is not always the case, but often is, and I attribute it to the mothers not being such good milkers as some other kinds. It seems to be their nature to run to fat rather than milk.

"I have no trouble in successfully breeding my Essex, and almost invariably find purchasers well satisfied, and thenceforth advocates of the breed.

"In my opinoin, though they may never become so popular as some, they will still be a valuable standard breed."

CHAPTER VIII.

YORKSHIRES.—CHESHIRES, OR JEFFERSON COUNTY SWINE, OF NEW YORK.—LANCASHIRES.—VICTORIAS.—NEAPOLITANS.—JERSEY REDS.—DUROCS.

The breeds of swine named above are so little known by the general farmers of the country, that such merits as they have are overlooked and neglected. Unlike the more prominent breeds, the information to be obtained respecting them is quite meagre.

We have been unable to find anything of much importance, or that would be deemed more authentic than the reports made to, and adopted by the National Convention of Swine Breeders, held at Indianapolis, November 20th, 1872.

YORKSHIRES.

We have never met in the West, at fairs or elsewhere, a distinct breed of swine known as Yorkshires, nor have we conversed with any one having any positive practical knowledge of them, but submit the report on this breed as presented to the Convention at Indianapolis:

Professor Jones, of Iowa; Jacob Kennedy, and I. N. Barker, of Indiana, in their Report on Yorkshires have the following:

* * * * "Their color and characteristics have been traced, in a greater or less degree, into every popular breed of swine which has been made up or attempted to be established as thorough-bred, either in the United States or England; indeed, we might say, into every breed, save the Essex, or Neapolitan, imported by Lord Western. These were the only pure bred black hogs of which we have any account, either in this country or the old. And we think it may safely be said of these white hogs, that they are the only pure and distinct breed of hogs or pigs, save the black, that are now bred on this continent. Do not understand us as contending that all black and all white hogs are thorough or pure bred; but that all breeds in this country of mixed colors are what their color indicates—are mixed or cross bred, hence not pure and distinct

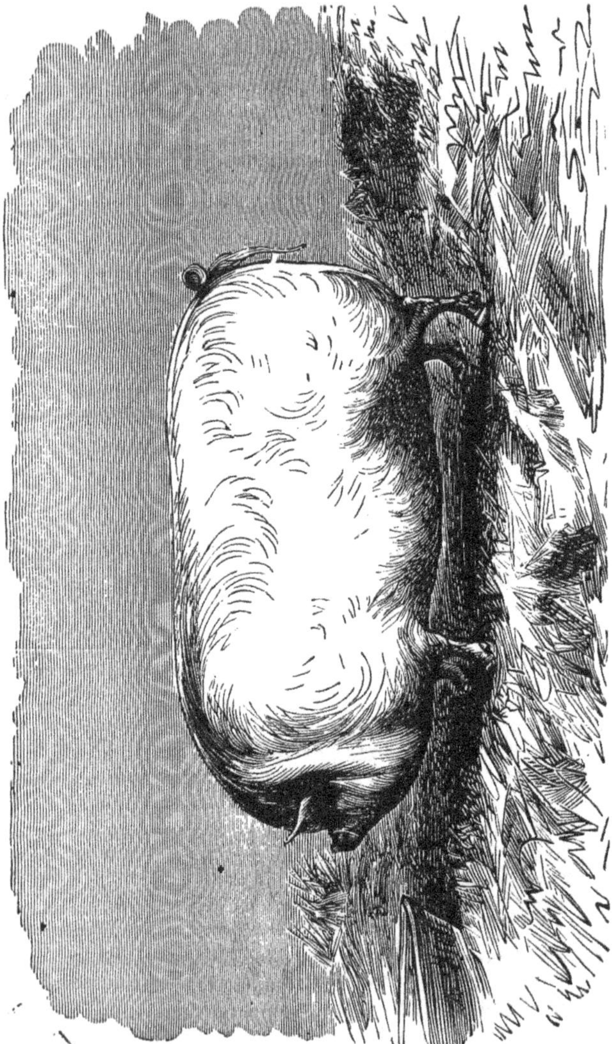

Fig. 6.—SMALL WHITE YORKSHIRE SOW.

very small, straight, and smooth, measuring below the knee but six inches in circumference. The surface of her body, jowl, and legs, was smooth, and free from ridges and creases, and well covered with a short, smooth coat of white hair. This, we think, might be taken as a fair description of all thorough-bred animals of this stock. It seems to be in this country, as it is said to be in England, in almost every way a middle breed. We know of no breed of hogs in this country but what might in some degree be improved by crossing occasionally with the thorough-bred Yorkshire, which has been bred pure in this country since 1860. We have seen whole neighborhoods and districts where the swine were nearly all lop-eared, rough-skinned, black, sandy, and spotted white or blue, where, in a few years, by introducing a few of these pure blooded white hogs, the general stock was made white, given erect ears, and skin made smooth. Such a result cannot be attained by Chester Whites alone, but it can be accomplished by the thorough-bred Yorkshire. They are so thorough-bred and positive that they carry their own color when crossed with almost any other breed, even if it is entirely black. Hence it is difficult to find a breed of swine in this age of their improvement, in which the white Yorkshire does not crop out in some particular. And again, the pure white Yorkshire and the black Essex, or Neapolitan, may be bred together in such a way as to duplicate the color of any other breed of hogs to be found among us. And hence we claim the white Yorkshire, as now established in this country and England, is the most thorough-bred hog known. The Yorkshires are the most valuable swine to breed from or to cross with that we have ever met with in this country; and for these reasons: 1. They are of a size, shape, and flesh, that are desirable for the family or the packer's use. 2. They have a hardy, vigorous constitution, and a good coat of hair protecting the skin so well, either in extreme cold or hot weather, that it rarely freezes or blisters. 3. They are very quiet, and good graziers; they feed well and fatten quickly at any age. 4. They are very prolific and good mothers, and the young never vary in color, and so little in shape that their form, when matured, may be determined in advance by an inspection of the sire and dam. This we have learned by a practical experience of many years in breeding, slaughtering, packing, and consuming.

"'The Yorkshire medium or middle breed,' in the words of Mr. Sydney, 'is a modern invention of Yorkshire pig-breeders, and perhaps the most useful and the most popular of the white breeds, as it unites, in a striking degree, the good qualities of the large and the small. It has been produced by a cross of the large and the small York and the Cumberland, which is larger than the small York. Like the large whites, they often have a few pale-blue spots on the skin, the hair on these spots being white. All white breeds have these spots more or less, and they often increase in number as the animals grow older. * * * *

"The middle Yorkshire breed are about the same size as the Berkshire breed, but have smaller heads, and are much lighter in the bone. They are better breeders than the small whites, but not so good as the large whites; in fact, they occupy a position in every respect between the two breeds. Hence their size can be increased or diminished without crosses with any other breed or color."

CHESHIRE, OR JEFFERSON COUNTY SWINE OF NEW YORK.

The following was adopted by the Swine Breeders' Convention, of 1872, as the report upon this breed:

"These hogs originated in Jefferson county, New York, and it is claimed by some of the breeders that they started from a pair of pigs bought of Mr. Woolford, of Albany, New York, which were called Cheshires. However that may be, there is no such distinct breed of hogs known as Cheshires, in England, and there is no record of any hogs of this name having been imported into this country.

"Yorkshires have been imported into Jefferson county from time to time, and the so-called Cheshires have been improved by crossing with their best hogs bought in Canada. Mr. A. C. Clark, of Henderson, was, for a number of years, a prominent breeder of these pigs, and he informed us that whenever he found a pig better than those he owned, he purchased it and crossed it upon his own stock. In this way this family of hogs have been produced, and they are now known and bred in many portions of the United States. Their breeding in Jefferson county has diminished during the last two or three years.

"They are pure white, with a very thin skin of pink color, with little hair; are not uniform in this respect, as pigs in the same litter differ widely in the amount of hair; the snout is often long, but very slender and fine; the jowls are plump and the ears erect, fine and thin; the shoulders are wide, and the hams full; the flesh of these hogs is fine-grained, and they are commended on account of the extra amount of mess pork in proportion to the amount of offal; the tails of the pigs frequently drop off when young."

Under date of April 11th, 1876, Col. F. D. Curtis (who made the foregoing report) writes the author: "There is nothing to add to the report. I do not know of but one breeder of these pigs in Jefferson county, N. Y., at the present time, who makes their breeding a specialty. There was never a connected effort to make them uniform, and thus establish a breed, and it was quite common, in our State, to call any cross of Yorkshires or Suffolks by the name of Cheshires.

"Mr. Clark, as long as he bred, bred to a standard, and I think Mr. Green, who is the leading breeder now, is trying to do the same thing."

Several breeders of fine stock, in Kentucky, and some of the Western States, have hogs that are called Cheshires, but we are doubtful of their being bred the same as the swine known by that name in New York, and the more Eastern States.

Knowing Mr. J. H. Sanders of Chicago, a well-known writer on live stock, had bred "Cheshires" somewhat extensively, and with success, in Iowa, we applied to him for some authentic information respecting them.

He replies: "In my opinion, the Cheshire is simply a derivative of the Yorkshire, as are also the Suffolk, Lancashire Short-face, Middle York, York-Cumberland, and all the other English breeds of white hogs. I bred the so-called Cheshires for six or seven years, and took a deep interest in noticing the variations and changes that were produced in that time by selection, in-breeding, and crossing. Within the space of seven years, without introducing any blood but what was supposed to be pure, I produced all the different types of the Yorkshire, from the large York, down to the Lancashire Short-face.

The white color was firmly fixed, and I never knew one of my Cheshire boars to get a pig that had a black hair on it, although they were bred to sows of all breeds, including the purest Essex. Another peculiarity that I watched with interest, was the frequent appearance of blue spots in the skin of the purest and best bred specimens. This peculiarity would sometimes disappear for one or two generations, and would again crop out stronger than ever.

"The type which I finally succeeded in fixing upon the Cheshires, as bred by me, was almost identical, in size, form, and quality, with the most approved medium Berkshire. Indeed, so marked was this resemblance in everything but color, that they were often facetiously called 'White Berkshires.'

"As bred by me, I regarded them as among the very best of white hogs.

"They were *well haired*, had a very delicate pink skin, and their meat was *most excellent, tender, and juicy.*"

VICTORIAS.

Mr. Charles E. Leland, of Albany, New York, submitted the following report at the Convention:

"The family of pigs known as Victorias originated with Col. Frank D. Curtis, Kirby Homestead, Charlton, Saratoga county, New York. They were made by crossing the Byfield hogs with the native, in which there was a strain of the Grazier. Subsequent crosses were made with the Yorkshire and Suffolk; the result being a purely white hog, of medium size. The name has no significance, unless it is intended as a compliment to the English Queen. These pigs, if pure bred, should have a direct descent from a sow called *Queen Victoria*, which may be said to be the mother of the family. She was pronounced, by good judges, to be almost perfect, and was the winner of a number of first prizes. Breeders in the Eastern States have long felt the need of a medium-sized white hog, with all the good points of the English breeds, without their objectionable features—a breed which would mature early, and be covered with a good coat of hair to protect it from the cold in winter and the heat in summer. Col. Curtis began breeding nearly twenty years ago to try and meet this want. At the fair of the New York State Agricultural Society, which was held at Elmira, he exhibited a sow, *Princess Alice*, and six pigs, which was the first

time the Victorias have been presented at a State fair for a competition with other swine. The first prize was awarded to the pigs, and the second to the sow.

"CHARACTERISTICS AND MARKINGS OF THE VICTORIAS.

"The color is white, with a good coat of fine soft hair; the head thin, fine, and closely set on the shoulders; the face slightly dishing; the snout short; the ears erect, small, and very light or thin; the shoulders bulging and deep; legs short and fine; the back broad, straight, and level, and the body long; the hams round and swelling, and high at the base of the tail, with plaits or folds between the thighs; the tail fine, and free from wrinkles or rolls; feathers or rosettes on the back are common; the skin is thin, soft, and elastic; the flesh fine-grained and firm, with small bone and thick side-pork. The pigs easily keep in condition, and can be made ready for slaughter at any age."

Since the foregoing was first printed a gentleman in Laporte county, Indiana, has made considerable progress in "inventing" and disseminating a family of swine which he has also named "Victorias"; but they are in every way distinct from those originated by Col. Curtis. They are medium-sized white swine of plain appearance, and in the hands of the originator have been quite successful at fairs and fat-stock shows. To obtain them he says he bred together Berkshires and Poland-Chinas, also Chester Whites and Suffolks, and then mated the offspring of these mixtures, which "has produced the model hog, guaranteed to reproduce itself white every time"!

NEAPOLITANS.

We have never seen a specimen of this breed, and are of the opinion that none of them are bred, at present, in this country, unless in the vicinity of New York. Their admitted influence in the improvement of English breeds, especially the Essex, in the hands of Lord Western and Mr. Fisher Hobbs, of Essex, England, make them of interest to fanciers of highly refined pigs.

Colonel M. C. Weld, of New York, submitted to the Swine Breeders' Convention a lengthy report on Neapolitans, from which we learn that the best specimens imported into this country came from near Naples, Italy, and that their earliest introduction was by Hon. James G. King, of Weehawken, N. J., in about 1840–41.

Some of these were pure black, others slate-color, some ash-colored, or a dirty-white, and others more or less spotted. About 1850, Wm. Chamberlain, of Red Hook, N. Y., imported some from Sorrento, Italy. These and some of their progeny were uniformly of a dark-slate color. Other parties, who had traveled in Italy, and been much pleased with the pork of Naples and the surrounding country, caused small stocks of these pigs to be imported for their own use; but few, if any of them, were offered for sale for breeding purposes.

It is believed by some, who knew them well, especially in England, that this breed has had an existence in the country about Naples for hundreds of years. Sidney's Youatt on the Pig says: "It is probable the Neapolitans are descendants of the dark Eastern swine imported by early Italian voyagers, and cultivated to perfection by the favorable climate and welcome food"; also that they are "black, or rather brown, with no bristles, and consequently delicate when first introduced into our northern climate."

About 1855, Dr. Phillips, of Memphis, Tennessee, obtained some pigs, bred from the Chamberlain importations. He found them more satisfactory than any of the numerous breeds he had tried, especially for using as a cross. In a letter to Col. Weld, he states that "the only objection to the breed is that the pigs are delicate, up to four or six months of age—after that they can live with he common hog."

Col. Weld has owned them imported direct from Italy, and thinks the fact that these pigs are almost hairless, has caused their reputation for delicacy, and that, treated as a high-bred race should be, they are not delicate, but quite the contrary, though he would not have them farrowed in winter, or in too close confinement. Their pork is described by A. B. Allen as being like "young, tender, fat chicken." They are classed with the small breeds.

The Convention adopted the following as the

"CHARACTERISTICS AND MARKINGS OF THE NEAPOLITANS.

"Head small; forehead bony and flat; face slightly dishing; snout rather long and very slender; ears small, thin, standing forward nearly horizontally, and quite lively; jowls very full; neck short, broad, and heavy above; trunk long, cylindrical, and well-ribbed back; back flat, and ribs arching, even in low flesh; belly horizontal on the lower line; hindquarters higher than the fore, but not very much so; legs very fine, the bones and joints being smaller than those of any other breed; hams and shoulders well developed and meaty; tail fine, curled, flat at the extremity, and fringed with hair on each side; general color slaty, or bluish-plum color, with a cast of coppery-red; skin soft and fine, nearly free from hair, which, when found upon the sides of the head and behind the forelegs, is black, and soft, and rather long; flesh firm and elastic to the touch."

JERSEY REDS.

The following is from the Report of the Convention:

"The positive origin of this family of Swine is unknown. They have been bred in portions of the State of New Jersey, for upwards of fifty years, and with many farmers are considered to be a valuable variety. They are of large size and capable of making a heavy growth, five hundred and six hundred pounds weight being common. Mr. David Pettitt, of Salem county, N. J., has known of these hogs for thirty years, and Mr. D. M. Brown, of Windsor, for nearly fifty years. They are now extensively bred in the middle and southern portions of New Jersey. In some neighborhoods they are bred quite uniform, being of a dark-red color, while in other sections they are more sandy, and often patched with white. They are probably descendants from the old importations of Berkshires, as there is no record of the Tamworth, the red hogs of England, ever having been brought into this country; nor is this likely, as the Tamworth were not considered a valuable breed, and were confined to a limited breeding. The Reds resemble the old Berkshires in many respects, but are now much coarser than the improved swine of this breed.

"CHARACTERISTICS.—A good specimen of Jersey Red should be red in color, with a snout of moderate length, large lop-ears, small head in proportion to the size and length of the body; they should be long in the body, standing high and rangy on thin legs; bone coarse; heavy tail and brush; hair coarse, including the bristles on the back. They are valuable on account of their size and strong constitution and capacity for growth. They are not subject to mange."

DUROCS.

These hogs have only a local reputation, and of them Col. F. D. Curtis reported to the Convention as follows:

"There is another family of heavy hogs called Duroc, which are bred in Saratoga county, New York, which are finer in the bone and carcass than the Reds. They have been bred, with their crosses, in this region of country, for about twenty years. They are very hardy, and grow to a large size."

Early in 1883 a number of breeders of so-called "red hogs" met at Elk Horn, Wis., and formed an organization to be known as the Duroc or Jersey Red Swine Club, with a view to advance the improvement of the breed, and establishing a registry of pedigrees. The standard agreed upon by the Club is as follows:

"The true Duroc or Jersey Red should be long, quite deep-bodied, not round, but broad on the back, and holding the width well out to the hips and hams. The head should be small, compared with the body, with the cheek broad and full, with considerable breadth between the eyes. The neck should be short and thick, and the face slightly curved, with the nose rather longer than in the English breeds; the ears rather large and lopped over the eyes and not erect. Bone not fine. nor yet coarse, but medium. The legs medium in size and length, but set well under the body and well apart, and not cut up high in the flank or above the knee. The hams should be broad and full well down to the hock. There should be a good coat of hair of medium fineness, inclining to bristles at the top of the shoulders; the tail being hairy and not small; the hair usually straight, but in some cases a little wavy. The color should be red, varying from dark, glossy, cherry red, and even brownish hair, to light yellowish red, with occasionally a small fleck of black on the belly and legs. The darker shades of red are preferred by most breeders, and this type of color is the most desirable. In disposition they are remarkably mild and gentle. When full grown they should dress from four hundred to five hundred pounds, and pigs at nine months old should dress from two hundred and fifty to three hundred pounds."

CHAPTER IX.

THE RELATIVE MERITS OF THE SUFFOLK, ESSEX, AND BERKSHIRE.

BY E. W. COTTRELL.

"The question is very often asked me by persons who are desirous of procuring some one of the improved breeds of swine, which of these three standard breeds do I consider best for the farmer, and it is a question which I find difficult to decide, even now, after quite an extensive experience of nearly six years with the three breeds side by side. I consider, however, that there is so little actual difference in the result, that fancy might guide the choice without serious detriment to one's judgment. Each, being a distinct and original breed, must have its own peculiarities and distinctive qualities, and the question to decide is, which of these qualities are most desirable, and which of the breeds possess and combine the most of them?

"Fancy must decide the question of beauty and appearance, and one person's judgment in that respect is as good as another's. Association with either for any length of time will generally occasion prejudice in its favor, and either breed possesses sufficient beauty to secure them hosts of admirers; and while I admire alike perfect specimens of either breed, I believe that the improved Berkshire displays a more majestic style and graceful appearance than any other of the swine species; there seems to be a stately bearing and royal mien, that I cannot help but admire as they move about the premises, and the contrast of the exact markings upon their beautiful black color adds another feature of beauty.

"In regard to the more essential question, however, of relative quality and profit, I will say that there are several things which must be taken into consideration, and one must choose those which combine the greatest number of desirable qualities for his purpose; that is, the object in view should decide the question. If the object is to produce a superior quality of delicious and wholesome pork, beautifully mixed with lean and fat, that is tempting and enjoyable from almost any part of the animal, I can safely recommend the Berkshire. They are also probably the most hardy of all the improved swine species; always healthy and thrifty, and generally docile and quiet in their natures, besides being very prolific, perhaps more so than any other of the improved breeds. The sows are invariably good milkers, and good mothers, one often successfully rearing from eight to twelve pigs.

"The improved also mature quite early, and at eight or nine months will give from two hundred to two hundred and fifty pounds of pork, and in many cases much more, with extra care. At eighteen months they will run from three hundred and fifty to four hundred and fifty pounds of pork each. We have had them weigh, at two years, seven hundred and eighty pounds, and not at all coarse or overgrown in style either. They are generally very uniform in every respect, though there are some families that attain a little more size than others. They are not ravenous like the common hog, but are good feeders, and what they eat seems to do them good all over; and, in fact, without discussing the subject further, they can be briefly summed up as a hardy, prolific, domestic, and reasonably easy-keeping animal, and one that can be sent to market at almost any age, with profit to the producer, and satisfaction to the consumer. Consequently, in my judgment, one who is undecided in his choice cannot go far astray in selecting the Berkshires.

"In summing up the desirable qualities which the Suffolks possess, however, we find them no less valuable, and perhaps even more profitable, for some purposes, than those of any other breed, unless we except the Essex. They are without question the earliest to mature, take on fat more readily, and produce more net pork with the same amount of feed than any other of the hog kind. These are certain facts, and very desirable ones when corn is worth eighty cents per bushel. Two pounds each per day is no uncommon average gain through the feeding season, and I have known an increase of three and one-half pounds per day for six weeks, or a total of one hundred and forty-seven pounds for one pig in six weeks time.

"And this propensity for fattening exists from the time they are sucklings; they can be fatted as well at six or eight months as at any other age; and this is a very desirable feature, for spring pigs can be sent to the market weighing two hundred and fifty pounds without much extra exertion, and the pork, rightly handled, will *always* bring a half-dollar, and perhaps more, per hundred than will the commoner kinds; and in reality it is worth much more to the consumer from the fact of its quality. The head and feet are almost nominal appendages, while the bones of the carcass are so fine and small that they cause but little loss.

"The objection is often raised that they are apt to be too fat for use, etc. Of course this is only from persons of superficial ideas. It might as well be said that sugar is too sweet, or vinegar too sour, especially when lard is eighteen cents per pound, and spare-ribs and other trimmings worth only four or five cents per pound. It is the fat that affords the greatest profit, and profit being the object, the animal which will produce the most fat, with the least expense, is the one for the purpose; and this animal is unquestionably the Suffolk, for they do certainly excel in this peculiarity, particularly at an early age. Notwithstanding the above facts, it should not be inferred that the pork is inferior as a meat for the table. The animal may have a surplus of fat, but the fleshy parts afford as delicate and wholesome table meat as can be found among the hog kind, and certainly as delicious. The trimmings from a dressed Suffolk will average but about ten per cent, while those from the long-legged, long-nosed, thick-skinned, coarse-boned kind, often make twenty per cent. The conclusions obtained from the above facts are obvious without farther comment, and I will now make reference to some of the other desirable features which the Suffolk possesses, a special one being their docile, quiet disposition. They are not inclined to stray if running loose, nor will they root up pastures and meadows if turned in upon them, even if not provided with rings; and they are seldom known to squeal or clamor, if half cared for. It is owing to this quiet, domestic nature that they grow and fatten so rapidly and economically. They also have a good constitution, and are invariably healthy with us, when past the tender age; also as hardy as any. As before stated, they are not ravenous, though good feeders, with a sharp appetite for what they require. When fed with regularity, they will be on hand at the usual time with almost exact promptness, and enter into the business of feeding with vigor, after which they will retire to their beds and attend wholly to business, which, for them, is to grow and fatten.

"The Essex are so very similar to the Suffolk, in nearly every respect except color, that the above description of qualities can be applied to them; perhaps they do not mature quite so early as the former, but they attain nearly as much weight, and fatten quite as easy, having the same quiet disposition and nature. Their skin, from its color, affords them one advantage over the Suffolks; that is, when the pigs of the latter are very young, if exposed to a burning sun, they are very liable to scald or blister upon the back, while this is never the case with the Essex. Here let me say that when Suffolk pigs are farrowed during the summer; or early fall, when the sun is strong, they should be protected from its scalding rays until five or six weeks of age. The Essex have as many good qualities as any other breed, and deservedly have a great many friends. In fact, a person cannot go far astray in selecting either of the three above breeds, and I am sure he will be satisfied with whichever kind his fancy may lead him to choose, after giving them a fair trial."

In writing of numerous experiments made by him, in crossing thorough-bred swine, Mr. Cottrell says:

"There is no question but the proper crossing of thorough-breds for a season will produce rapid and profitable pork-makers, but there seems to be some difference of opinion, and a great lack of information in general, among farmers and breeders, as to the crosses that produce the best results.

"The very best results we have ever obtained from any cross of thorough-breds, was that of the Suffolk upon the Essex. One case, which was almost a marvel, I will give for example. It is that of a litter which was farrowed the 16th day of March, and fed from the following 1st of October until the 24th of December, which made them nine months and eight days old when killed. The weight of the largest one was 402, and not one of them weighed less than 300. The pigs run upon the farm, being kept in a growing and thriving condition until October, when we took them up and forced them along, as the result shows.

"This marked improvement upon either breeds in the first cross is probably the result of uniting their excellent characteristics, which seem to be more fully developed, and stronger, than in either original. It is a fact, at least, that the feeding and maturing qualities are more or less improved in the cross. Neither is the style or beauty lost in the cross, for the symmetry and proportion are still retained. The color is generally black and white; sometimes one pig will be either all black or all white, but usually they are sheeted—that is, each spread in large patches, and very distinct. It is very seldom that we see a 'speckled' pig among thorough bred crosses; there is generally a foreign mixture when they occur. One peculiar feature with the color of this cross is, that invariably the black is in excess upon the hind part of the animal, while the white will predominate upon its fore parts. I have seen them one-half pure black and the other half pure white, with the dividing line where the colors meet forming a circle around the body at the middle. The peculiar marking makes quite an attractive contrast.

"We also found that the Berkshire and Essex make an excellent cross for feeding purposes. As a principle, I do not consider it advisable to cross the improved Berkshire with any other, on their own account, but prefer rather to keep that breed distinct and up to the mark by occasionally renewing with a foreign blood of its own kind. By foreign blood, I mean that of a distant or unrelated family. They are a standard breed, very near perfection in themselves, possessing qualities that cannot be very much improved upon without affecting the combination that constitutes the Berkshire, and stamps them with a character wholly their own, and which only requires to be kept to the ideal of their style and perfection to satisfy the requirements of almost every class, condition, and locality. The true well bred Berkshire has the stamp of the thorough-bred, and possesses the merits required for its purpose, and great pains should be taken to perpetuate the purity of that blood. However, when it is necessary or advisable to cross them, it should be made with the Essex, whenever practicable. The result of a single cross will always give satisfaction, the produce being such as will feed quick and mature sooner than the pure bred Berkshire, and the pork is second to none that goes to market. The general style and appearance of the animals will be similar, except in the markings; some will be more or less spotted, some marked like the Berkshire, some partially marked, and some all black. This cross, continued upon itself, will lose its identity with either breed, and eventually will result in a lot of mongrels.

"Upon the common kinds the Berkshire will do much good, and bring out a great improvement, but is not equal to the Suffolk or Essex in this respect. Of course, there are other breeds which will improve the common hog, but I know of none to be compared to the three above mentioned, from the fact of their being pure and standard breeds, that have come down in the same line for generations, and established distinct qualities and characteristics that are transmitted from one generation to another with as much exactness and certainty as can be found in any class of the animal kind. And the fact that they are capable of stamping upon their progeny the desirable points they possess, and reproduce themselves, as it were, with almost a positive certainty, is what gives them such great value as improvers of our stock.

"I have said that I believe certain crosses of the thorough-breds to be superior to either of the full bloods, for feeding purposes. The question may be asked, why not continue the breeding from these crosses?

"The fact is this, as I have before stated, after the first cross, the identity of the breed is lost, and with it the power to transmit its particular type is correspondingly reduced, and by continuing in the same line we lose all trace of the original. By using a thorough-bred upon the cross, of course, we produce equally as good results each time. For feeding purposes, and by a continuation of this practice, a superior class of pork-makers will always be obtained.

"And so, if one has a number of breeding sows of the common sort, let him procure a thorough-bred male, and I will guarantee that the result of the first cross will pay all the cost. But because a lot of very good animals has been obtained from this course, do not select your next male breeder from them, or the good already gained will be lost. But continue to use a thorough-bred male upon the produce, and those that have not tried it before will wonder at the rapid improvement of their stock, and why they have been so long behind the age of improvement and advancement."

RAISING AND FATTENING SWINE.

CHAPTER X.

THE BOAR—HOW TO CHOOSE, AND HOW TO KEEP HIM.

To claim that success in swine-breeding depends upon the proper selection of a boar, might not be wholly correct, but it is safe to say that many failures in the business have been in a large degree due to mistakes made at the beginning in the choice of breeding animals, especially males.

However good the sows of a herd may be, the good qualities of the stock quickly deteriorate if inferior boars are used, while, on the other hand, the offspring of inferior sows can be rapidly improved in form and quality, by using well bred boars.

It is no longer disputed by persons familiar with the principles of improved breeding, that the male parent mostly determines the outward form and structure, while the female chiefly determines the internal structure of the offspring, a somewhat striking illustration of which is afforded in the breeding together of an ass and a mare, the produce of which is a mule, and the mule is essentially, with slight modifications, an *ass*. A she ass bred to a stallion, produces the hinny, which is essentially a modified *horse*, the mule and the hinny each having the outward form, muscular structure, locomotive organs, and voice of its sire.

Assuming that these premises are correct, it must be apparent to the breeder and farmer, that the judicious selection of a boar is of prime importance, and that success is not assured in this branch of his business without it.

Among the prominent characteristics of the boar should be a fine external form, which is the result of a superior internal organism ; a short, broad face, with round heavy under jaw, and thick, short neck, indicate strong vitality and assimilating powers, two functions requisite in every first-class, meat-producing animal; width between the fore legs, and large girth immediately behind them, denotes room for large and active lungs, the very foundation of any animal. Ribs that are long and well sprung outward from the back, show capacity of stomach. The broad loin and well developed ham are signs of active kidneys. A clean, fine, and elastic skin, covered with soft, lively hair, free from bristles, denotes a healthy liver, and freedom from internal fever. A fine muzzle and limbs, clean, small joints, and standing square up on the feet, denote solidity, strength, and firmness of the animal's framework; while the dished, or concave face, and slightly drooping ear, are unerring signs of an easy keeper, and a quiet, contented disposition.

These are some of the features demanded in a good boar, and such an animal in perfect condition will not be sluggish and clumsy, but have a lively animated appearance, and move about freely and nimbly, unless kept in too close confinement on too much fattening food.

The herd, or family of hogs from which it is designed to select a boar, should be closely scanned, and if the animals show uniformity of breeding, good forms and constitutions, with even feeding qualities, it is a safe one to select breeders from; on the other hand, the weedy herd, wherein no two animals are alike, should be given a wide berth.

It is essential to choose a boar in some measure with reference to the style of females it is desired to cross him on, with a view to having deficient points in the sows corrected by the boar in the offspring. Should the sows be light in the ham or shoulder, the boar should be especially good there ; sows inclined to be razor-backed, should be bred to a boar with broad back, and well sprung ribs. If the sows are too coarse about the legs, neck, head, and ears, attention should be paid to securing a boar with short neck, fine ear, dish face, fine bone, and heavy jowls. If too "light and airy," too far from the ground, too active, too restless and uneasy, the opposite should be prominent characteristics of the boar. He should, in a majority of cases, be selected from a family or strain that is, and should himself be, somewhat smaller and more compact than animals upon which he is to be crossed, and in the swine herd, as in all domestic stock, constitution is of prime importance, and no animal without broad and deep fore-quarters has it.

He should be pure, of such breed as the owner may deem best, for if not pure, he cannot be depended on to stamp his own qualities on his offspring, as none but thorough-breds will invariably do so. The boar of mixed and unknown breeding is to be shunned as a snare and a delusion. If the Berkshires or a Berkshire cross is preferred, a pure Berkshire boar should be used. If the Essex seems most desirable, use a pure Essex boar; or if the Poland-China cross promises the best results, use a pure Poland-China boar. Do the same with any breed that may be preferred, and success is certain; but to use a boar that is a mixture of several breeds, however pure they may individually be, is to progress backward.

It is an undeniable fact, that many who pay a liberal price to obtain a boar that suits them, afterward treat him in such a way that they derive but small benefit from the investment. One of the two most common modes of mistreatment is, to confine him in a close pen, where he is deprived of exercise and fed upon the richest and most fattening food the establishment affords: lack of activity and of virility are the results. The other mode is, to turn him with an unlimited number of sows, gilts, and stock hogs, to fight, and fret, and tease, until he becomes the shabbiest, the most ungainly, unthrifty hog on the place.

Either of these extremes must be avoided, and a more rational method pursued, or the best results cannot be secured. While too close confinement is bad, it is not so bad as to allow a boar to roam at will among the other hogs of a farm, where he is as much out of place as a stallion would be if turned loose with a herd of horses. He should be kept in a comfortable pen, with a lot or pasture adjoining, and supplied with a variety of nutritious food, which means something more than dry corn, with an occasional drink of diluted dish-water. His condition should always be that of thrift, and vigorous health, not too fat, nor yet so lean that as a barrow he would be considered unfit for pork. If too fat, he will be clumsy, slow, and in no wise a sure getter. As to the age at which he should begin service, we have, after considerable observation and experience, come to the conclusion that it is unwise to permit the boar to be with a sow at all until at least seven months old, and then only in exceptional cases and very sparingly. Immature sires cannot be expected to generate vigorous progeny. At a year old, moderate service will not injure him, and properly kept, he should be at his best as a sire, when from eighteen months to five years old, when he is matured and developed, and has every advantage over a half-grown immature pig; the finest, strongest litters are invariably obtained from large old sows, bred to aged boars.

We well understand that it is of little use to recommend farmers, who raise or purchase fine boar pigs, to keep them until a year and a half or two years old, before using them, as not one in ten thousand would do so, yet those who properly keep their boars that length of time, will find the value of their breeding greatly enhanced. Aged boars are generally looked upon as unpleasant animals to keep, especially if they have become vicious and disposed to use their tusks—a view in which the author himself shares somewhat—but they are certainly less dangerous and troublesome than the gentlest bull or stallion, while, of course, none of them are desirable, or intended for, household pets or door-yard ornaments.

A pen or fence sufficiently high and strong to restrain the other hogs of the farm, cannot be depended on to keep the boar in his place, and if opportunity offers, he will soon become unruly; consequently, it is much the best to keep him, from the first, in an enclosure which will afford him no practice in the art of breaking out.

If his quarters are isolated from those of other hogs, especially sows, and sow pigs—some of which are likely to be in heat most of the time—he will usually be quiet and gentle,—in fact, a pretty well behaved hog, though much depends upon his natural disposition, and more upon the treatment given him.

With a fair chance, some of the first litters will enable his owner to judge of his merits as a sire, which, if satisfactory, will make it worth while to keep him for several seasons. Unless certain of doing very much better, we would not hesitate to breed him to his own pigs, even though we consider indiscriminate in-and-in breeding as reprehensible in the extreme. We advise even this cross, *only* when the parents are both healthy, and it is desired to fix and retain in the offspring certain points, or qualities, that are of great value, and prominent in both boar and sow. Turned with a sow in heat until one service is given, she will have as many, and as good pigs as there would be if the boar was permitted to chase and worry her for three days and nights. The most experienced breeders concede this, and many will not allow but a single service.

It is safe to say that the bulk of the hog crop is produced by farmers who breed less rather than over a dozen sows, on an average, at any one season of the year. To keep a matured boar in the best condition, is felt to be quite an expense by one man who has but a few sows, and where three or four farmers live in proximity to each other, we think it much the best and cheapest plan for them to jointly own and keep one strictly good boar, instead of each keeping, wholly at his own expense, one that he thinks will do, though not so good as he would like, if the first cost and subsequent expense and trouble were less.

Properly managed, one boar would, in many cases, answer every purpose as well as a half dozen, for that number of small farmers, and if his cost and keep were shared by all, it would scarcely be felt, and at the same time the temptation to use some mongrel, or immature pig, would be removed.

Among the benefits resulting from this method would be, the use of a good boar, matured, and fitted for good service; an improved class of pigs, and a generous rivalry, encouraging each of his owners to keep a better grade of sows, under improved and more profitable conditions.

In sparsely settled neighborhoods, or where too many sows were to be bred, it would not be so practicable; but where possible, it would be a little of that much-talked-of "coöperation among farmers," which, when really practised, as well as preached, will indeed be found one of the touchstones of success.

When the time arrives for him to be superseded as the head of the herd, and it is desired to make him a barrow, it can be done by one active man operating as follows: After drawing up one hind leg, and fastening it securely to a post, or stake, fasten another rope around the upper jaw, back to the tusks, draw it tightly, and fasten it to another stake; in this position the animal can offer no serious resistance. The cut should be low down, and as small as possible; the low cut will afford a ready means of escape for all extraneous matter, and allow the wound to keep itself clean, there being no sack, or pocket, left to hold the pus formed during the healing process. It is not best to perform this operation when the boar is very fat, or the weather too warm, as the risk is much greater. If castrated early in the season, and kept on grass during the summer, the flesh, when he is made fat, will be but little more rank than that of other hogs. Kept with other hogs, if quarrelsome, there is danger of his doing them great injury with his tusks, and hence it is desirable to fatten a stag hog by himself. It is at this period that the old boar's true proportions will show themselves, as he will take on fat very rapidly, and present a greatly improved appearance; but when sold, the buyer will quite probably insist on paying for the "stag" only two-thirds the price of other hogs, which, in many cases, we have considered entirely too great a deduction.

CHAPTER XI.

THE SOW AND HER PIGS.

The measure of success attained by those who raise hogs, depends in no small degree upon the judicious selection, for breeding purposes, of sows that are best calculated, in their form, and general make up, to give birth to, and to nourish for several weeks, a reasonable number of well-formed, thrifty, vigorous pigs. The sow is the laboratory, wherein are developed the germs of the future herd, and, other things being equal, it is plain that this laboratory, or, if we may so call it, this machine-shop, must, to furnish the best results, be as near perfection as possible. She should be selected from a stock, or family, in which fertility is a characteristic; for this essential quality is hereditary, though lacking in numerous strains of the various breeds. The most promising pig at six or eight weeks, may fall far short of being so promising at six or eight months; and, for this reason, where it is practicable, it is better to defer the selection of sows for breeding purposes, until they have made considerable growth, and exhibit prominently certain characteristics which they should possess, and enable the breeder to form a more nearly correct judgment as to what their forms will be when they have matured.

At this time, she should appear to be of a form known as "rangy," *i. e.*, the opposite of compact, of loose and open build, long, yet quite broad on the back, with short neck and head, fine ear, heavy jowl—sure indications of an easy keeper, wide between the fore legs, deep sides, and heavy hams, well let down on the gambrel joint. She should be large and roomy, (in some respects rather the opposite of the boar), from healthy stock, a greedy feeder, and of great vitality, as indicated by large girth back of the fore legs, and a robust appearance generally. Coarseness is allowable in the sow, much more than in the boar, especially if she has great room for carrying a large litter, with indications of being a good suckler, as shown by having at least twelve prominent, well developed teats, or "dugs." The venerable Paschall Morris, of Philadelphia, one of the oldest and most intelligent breeders and improvers of swine in the United States, wrote: "I have always found that a hog with a dish-face, short nose, small head, and wide between the eyes, is an easy, quiet feeder. On the other hand, a long, large head, indicates, in a general way, a hard, uneasy feeder, and a great consumer."

Sows, well kept, will, in some cases, come in heat when not more than three months old; but, in all such cases, care should be taken to keep them separated from, or out of reach of, any boar pigs on the place. Eight months is as young as it is judicious or proper to breed them, and we would much prefer to have them a year old before letting to the boar. In all breeds, and especially those noted for early maturity, the vitality of the young animal is taxed to its utmost in making a rapid and vigorous growth, and to impose upon it, at the same period, the further burden of production, tends to make a failure of both. The sow not being matured, it is unnatural to expect the perfection in the offspring that the dam may possess; nature is, at the same time, perfecting the undeveloped mother, and promoting the growth of the young, and the result is, that both are losers, and deficient at maturity, and the mother can never recover from this division and deficit of nature's work.

A comparison of the litters from matured sows, with those of others, that were mere pigs themselves when bred, will furnish a practical illustration of this; the pigs from the large old sows, will be more in number, and frequently double the size of the others, at a month old; and with the same care, they will not unfrequently weigh 50 per cent. more, at nine or twelve months old. For this reason, sows that have proven themselves extra valuable as breeders and sucklers, should be retained as among the prized animals of the farm.

Those who pursue the plan of obtaining but one litter from a sow, and then converting her into pork, can never compete for size, style, and vigor, with those who raise stock from vigorous sows, from eighteen months to six years old.

Usually, when not with pig, or suckling, a sow will be in heat about three days out of twenty-one, or once in three weeks, and when she is to be bred, she should be free from fever, her system cooled and cleansed by a variety of food and loosening slops.

There can be no doubt that many valuable sows have been utterly ruined for breeding purposes, by over-feeding on corn and meal, which, alone, possess too much heat-producing and too little bone and muscle-forming material to supply the needs of the animal economy. On this account, sows should not be allowed to run with fattening hogs kept on corn, but in pasture, and allowed a plenty of slop, made of equal parts of shorts, corn meal, and wheat bran.

The main crop of pigs should come in the warm days of April, and that it may be so, sows should be bred as near the middle of December as may be ; though in the States not too far north, and where the best of care can be furnished at farrowing time, December 1st is not too early for old sows, and December 10th for young sows. Old sows will carry their pigs 112 or possibly 115 days, and young sows will sometimes farrow their first litter in from 100 to 106 days from the date of service.

It is generally believed among breeders, that a sow turned to the boar on the first symptoms of heat, will have mostly *sow* pigs, and that if she is not served until the period of heat is about passed, she will have mostly *boar* pigs.

While carrying her pigs, plenty of exercise, generous supplies of not too rich food, with comfortable quarters, are indispensable to success, and must not be overlooked. To allow sows to run among cattle, horses, or colts, exposes them in various ways to injuries that may cause the loss of valuable litters, especially if the sows are heavy and awkward.

It is bad policy to have sows fat at the time of taking the boar, as there are few cases in which a sow, thin in flesh, approaching to leanness, at that time, does not do better than one that is fat, or in what is called respectable show condition. After getting with pig, a sow fattens very readily, and if fed too much strong food, is likely to become pork-fat, have smaller pigs, and do badly in farrowing.

As the time approaches for the pigs to appear, the sow should be separated from any other hogs, and placed in a sheltered, yet sunny pen, provided with some short hay or straw, out of which she will arrange her nest. If given a large quantity of bedding, she will make her nest too deep, forming a sort of pit, into which the pigs will roll, and surely be crushed. A shallow nest is much the best, and many fine pigs, sometimes even whole litters, have been lost by giving the sow a too generous supply of bedding material. In warm weather, but little, if any, need be given, and in cold weather, the nest should be thoroughly protected on the outside, and made so comfortable that a great pile of hay or straw will not be necessary to prevent the pigs from becoming chilled. About six or eight inches from the floor, and the same distance from the sides of the pen, near the nest, a scantling, rail, or pole, should be fastened ; this will prevent the sow from crushing the little pigs between herself and the wall.

A sow well fed at the time of pigging, will usually lie more quietly, and endanger her pigs less by frequently getting up and lying down, than a hungry one. Sometimes young or small sows appear to be in so much misery, that they cannot be quiet, but if they have been petted and kindly treated, they will allow an attendant to remove the pigs as fast as they come, which may be the means of saving many of them that might otherwise be crushed or trampled to death.

Many good farmers have been aggravated beyond measure, by finding a favorite brood-sow in the act of destroying her litter of choice pigs, and none but those who have had such bitter experience, can realize how discouraging it is. My ideas on this subject are so nearly identical with those of Mr. A. C. Moore, the well-known breeder of Poland-Chinas, that I will use his own language to express them :

"The first losses of our litters are enormous. By improper care of the sow, and unsuitable places and surroundings for littering, many persons yearly sacrifice their gains in swine growing. Costiveness and its attendant evils, are among the impelling causes of ferocity in the sow. 'Coles Diseases of Domestic Animals' says it is because they are kept from earth, coal, ashes, etc., and advises allowing them as much room as possible, feeding them fresh earth, grass, sod, rotten wood, charcoal, ashes, etc., and says, after pigging, 'feed light, on light food for a few days,' and I wish to *emphasize* this last quotation. This applies, of course, more particularly to animals that have been kept on board floors. I do not believe that a sow will devour her young unless extremely costive, amounting almost to a state of frenzy—though having done so once, she may repeat the act without being in that condition. Breeding sows should not be allowed to run together in the same yard when pigs are expected; the taste of blood seems infectious, and opportunities often occur when costive animals will begin by eating dead pigs, or first destroy part of another's litter, and are thereby led to afterwards destroy their own.

"Don't do *too much* for them just before littering, and feed nothing but thin slop for three or four days after. * * * With quiet, proper feed, and a little care of some one at the proper time, a very small per cent will be lost in breeding. Insist on everything and everybody being quiet about your breeding pens."

When we find a sow destroying her pigs, or showing a disposition to do so, we saturate a small woolen cloth with kerosene, and carefully moisten the hair of the pigs with it, but are cautious to not get much of it on their tender skins—and we usually find that the kerosene dressing spoils the sow's relish for raw pig.

The feverish condition of the sow at farrowing time, will cause thirst, and a plenty of fresh water should be kept within her reach, notwithstanding the fact that she is being kept on sloppy food, as this will not prevent her needing water, any more than a person's having soup at meal-time will prevent his wanting water. For making a plenty of healthful milk, skimmed milk, wheat bran, and shorts mixed, are most excellent, and no careful breeder, anxious to do the best by his litters of pigs, should neglect to have a supply accessible for use when his sows are suckling. We have had very favorable results from feeding chopped (coarsely ground) rye, soaked from 24 to 36 hours, but not allowed to become too sour before feeding and consider it as near perfection in the way of a succulent, nutritious mess, for a sow suckling a number of greedy, growing pigs.

For the first weeks of a pig's life, the mother's milk is its drink as well as food, and therefore, in caring for suckling sows, it should be the aim to so feed them, that the largest possible quantity of milk, of only medium richness, will be furnished, instead of a limited supply of that which is extremely rich, the latter being less healthful, and more liable to cause fever, cough, constipation, and unsatisfactory growth.

Grass, or other green food, is not to be omitted from the bill of fare, and Red Clover is the standard green crop for swine, though Blue Grass (*Poa pratensis*) is by some considered preferable, but either is most excellent. It is difficult to satisfactorily manage the pasturing of several sows with pigs in the same field, on account of the larger pigs stealing from, and robbing the smaller ones of their share of milk, causing them to become stunted and very uneven in size. The only remedy is to separate them.

When pigs are three weeks old, they will usually begin to eat, if suitable food is placed where they can get it, and a small trough should be placed in a part of the pen or lot, inaccessible to the sow, and into this about three or four times a day, for several days, a little sweet milk can be poured—whatever they will drink up clean, but not more, increasing the quantity as they grow older, when some shelled corn, soaked in water twenty-four hours, or more, should be given, and, if convenient, sour milk, corn-meal mush, scalded bran with shorts, and such nourishing food as will make them a healthful variety.

Mr. Mooro, before quoted in this chapter, has probably handled with success as many pigs as any man living, and gives in his *Swine Journal* the following as his method of feeding them :

"My mode of feeding young pigs is to provide sufficient board floor, sheltered from the hot sun and the storms, on which to place the feed troughs. In these I feed shelled corn, soaked in barrels sunk in the ground, or bins; corn is soaked from 24 to 48 hours, owing to the weather. With the water that has soaked the corn, I make up a slop of ground oats and corn, mixed with bran and shorts from the mill. This slop, and the corn, is distributed to all the troughs, by means of buckets—those for the corn having holes in the bottom, to allow escape of water. From the troughs where the pigs are fed, I exclude the sows by means of bars that will let the pigs pass in and out of the trough, yard, or pen. I feed the sows on an adjoining floor, in similar troughs. Thus, pigs that are weaned, and such as are yet suckling, but large enough to take care of themselves, are fed from the same troughs. Of course, my younger pigs, from two to four weeks old, are fed in the stye with the sow—have a separate trough if necessary, and are not turned into a herd until they know their dam, and will suckle only at home; but with all the time and care we can give to the "training" of young pigs, there will be some thieves in the yards who will steal from another dam when they can get a good chance.

"All feed troughs must have strips nailed across the top, to partition off the feeding room of each pig. * * * In feeding, each pig must have a fair chance for its share; you should not pour swill into one end of a trough and calculate that a portion of your pigs will get their supply from the other end. Notice, and you will see that the big ones are always near the spout or first end—they have learned where the best swill is to be had, while the pigs at the further end—the little ones—are compelled to take the leavings as it runs to them, and are thus made themselves into "leavings." Pigs should never be fed on the ground when it is dusty or muddy.

"Though I have no doubt but that cooked or steamed food will amply pay for the cost and labor of preparation, I have never used it."

While believing that they should have as much corn as they will eat, it is very essential to their rapid growth, that other and softer food be supplied, making a variety that will be easily digested, and assist to keep their appetites sharp.

The boar pigs may be castrated when from two to eight weeks old, that they may recover from its effects before weaning time, and at that age, if help is not at hand, it can easily be done by a single person after a little practice. With the pig standing on his head in a nail keg, or something of similar size and shape, which confines him so closely as to prevent much troublesome resistance, the operation may be easily performed. If flies are troublesome, it is well to pour some kerosene into and over the wound. A preparation sold in the markets as "Frazer's Axle Grease," is an excellent salve for these and similar wounds and sores on any kind of stock, but if flies are not about, we do not use even this, and never had a pig die or do badly from being castrated.

Sows should be spayed when somewhat older, say at three months, and there are probably a thousand men who can do a tolerable job at castrating a boar, to one that is competent to properly spay a sow; unless it can be done by a person understanding it, it is risky business. We have seen an ignoramus ruin a herd of Berkshire shotes by spaying them in the belly in such a manner that, when they healed up, their bellies dragged on the ground.

Considerable observation leads us to the conclusion, that the only proper place to spay is in the side, and not there, unless by an expert. Where there is a probability of doing, or having it done successfully, we think it extremely desirable, as no hogs keep easier, or fatten better, than sows that have been properly spayed. (The reader will find this subject treated by one of the most successful and practical veterinary surgeons in the country, in the succeeding chapter.)

Weaning is a severe ordeal to many pigs, but those cared for, and taught to eat some weeks before, do not, as a rule, appear to have their growth noticeably checked, while others, that have depended entirely on the mother's milk, seem to have their growth entirely suspended, sometimes for many weeks.

As to the proper time for weaning, the owner must, to

some extent, be governed by surrounding circumstances. Sometimes it is necessary to wean when the pigs are five or six weeks old, and in other cases there may be no particular reasons for doing so until ten, or sometimes twelve weeks old; but at from seven to ten weeks old, most pigs are fit to be put away from the sows. If they cannot be successfully weaned at that age, it is difficult to say when they could be. Some pigs are really older at seven weeks than others at ten, and are better fitted for weaning.

Nothing is so well calculated to make them grow as a bountiful supply of sow's milk, and the pigs that have a plenty of other feed, with the milk of a well-slopped sow, for eight or ten weeks, will invariably have much the start in growth of those weaned at five or six weeks, no matter how much food and attention the earlier weaned pigs may have had.

If from the tendency of a sow to get too fat, or from other causes, she is bred the third or fourth day after farrowing, it is best to wean by the time the pigs are six weeks old, in order that their longer sucking may not injuriously affect the succeeding litter. If they have been accustomed to eating milk, grain, and grass, while running with the sow, this can be done without perceptibly checking their growth ; but otherwise, the sudden change not infrequently retards it for several weeks. It should not be forgotten, that with swine, as with all other stock, warmth is to a certain extent equivalent to food, for which reason comfortable shelter and clean, dry bedding, have a money value, as with these, they not only consume less food, but grow much faster.

The sow, in most cases, will take the boar from the second to the fourth day from farrowing, and if she is not served then, or fails to get with pig, she will not, as a general thing, breed again until the pigs have been weaned from two to four weeks—if not too much suckled down, in about three weeks.

It is not a good plan to take all the pigs from the sow, unless one or two of them can be turned with her some hours after, to draw out the milk she will have at that time, and again, say after a lapse of twenty-four hours. The way preferred by us is, to leave about two of the smallest with her for four or five days, and after that, leave only one for two or three days more, by which time the flow of milk will have been so gradually diminished, that no injury will result to the sow by keeping them entirely away from her.

After weaning pigs, the pasture is a good place for the sow, and if a mess of good slop is given her once a day, it will be fed to good advantage. When bred again, she should be so fed and cared for, as to gain something in flesh every day, and yet not become loaded down with fat from the use of too much heating and concentrated food. If treated in a friendly way, she will be friendly and well disposed, and ordinarily come as near paying richly for all she gets, as any animal kept on the farm.

CHAPTER XII.

CASTRATING AND SPAYING.

The necessity of castrating the boar pigs, for pork-making purposes, is generally admitted, but the importance of spaying such sow pigs, on the farm or in the herd, as are not designed for breeders, has never been appreciated as it should, or as it is likely to be, when the rearing of swine is conducted on such business principles as its importance demands. Open sows, running with other stock hogs, are a source of great annoyance, and where more than two or three are kept, there is scarcely a time when some one of their number is not in heat, and continually chasing the others, thus keeping them in a worried, fevered condition, extremely prejudicial to growth or fattening.

If all are neatly trimmed, this is avoided, the hogs are quiet and restful, and much time, trouble, and feed are saved.

All feeders agree, that no animals in the swine-herd feed more kindly and profitably, than spayed sows, and there are no buyers who would not as soon, or sooner, have them than barrows, when they would not buy a lot of open sows at any price. An open sow, when fat, of the same dimensions externally as a spayed sow or barrow, generally weighs from ten to twenty pounds less.

To the feeder, the buyer, or the butcher, unspayed sows are usually, in one way or another, a cheat, as they may weigh more than they are worth by having a litter of pigs in them, or may be utterly destitute of inside fat, from having recently suckled pigs; in either case they are of less value than their appearance would indicate. Spayed sows are not troublesome to their mates, are as good as they look for feeding or marketing, and command in all markets such prices as are paid for none but first-class stock.

There is no subject connected with the live stock interests, upon which so little has been written, or upon which it seems so difficult to get reliable information or directions, as this. In view of this want, we have had the following practical and explicit directions prepared by one of the most experienced and successful veterinary surgeons in the country, Dr. T. C. Miles, of Charleston, Illinois, whose practice in this branch of his profession is very extensive. Doct. M. says:

"As to the *time* for castrating boars, I would say, do it whenever most convenient, and the best *way* is the way understood by every old farmer, unless the hog is ruptured, in which case the striffen around the seed (called the scrotal sack) should be taken out with the seed, and the seed-string tied within the neck of the scrotal sack with a small twine. When this is done, cut off the seed-sack, and all behind the tie, and let the hog go. I do not like sewing up, as large tumors sometimes result from so doing. Should maggots develop in the gash where a hog has been cut, apply either turpentine or butter-milk.

"TO CASTRATE A RIDGLING HOG.

"In a ridgling hog, the seeds are not in a scrotal sack, or in their proper place, but in the body of the animal, immediately behind the kidneys.

"He should be cut in the side, the same as in spaying a sow, but the incision should be made of sufficient size to admit the whole hand, when the seeds can be found and easily pulled out.

"TO SPAY SOWS.

"One man should be in the pen to catch, and two to hold the sow, by the feet alone, flat on the ground on her right side, and stretched out tightly. The spayer, kneeling at the sow's back, will cut the hair off of the place where the incision is to be made, (a little back of the last rib, and about midway up and down); then cut a gash—if on a hundred-pound shote, about half an inch deep and three inches long, up and down; slip the flesh back each way, about an inch, making a round gash or wide incision; then turn the knife, and stick the blade straight in, gently, deep enough to go through the peritoneal lining, or inside striffen, at the upper corner of the incision. Then put the left fore-finger in, and with it and the right fore-finger, tear the hole large enough to allow working room for the fingers; feel inside near the back, with the first two fingers of the left hand, for the 'pride,' a little knotty lump, which cannot be mistaken, for there are no others like it within reach, but if it is not found—

as is sometimes the case, then feel for small guts, called the 'pig-bag,' and take them out the best you can, until the first 'pride' is reached; take this off; follow back down the pig-bed to a fork where two guts coming together form a larger one, as two branches running together form a creek; here take up the other branch until the lower 'pride' is reached; take it off, put the pig-bed back in good order, and see that it is all in the belly proper, and not left at the gash.

"Slack up the upper hind leg, so as to close the gash, and sew up with two stitches, taking good hold, but going only skin-deep; one stitch near the middle of the gash, the other above it; draw the edges together, so as to touch from the middle of the gash upward. Both stitches may be taken before tying either, and then tie the threads or twine, crossing each other, in the form of a letter X, and when the sow is let go, press the hand over the gash as she starts off.

"For spaying purposes, the thread or twine used should not be too harsh or too tightly twisted."

CHAPTER XIII.

PASTURE AND SUMMER FOOD.

The necessity of providing swine with summer pasture and green food, is, even in the best corn-producing districts, becoming more and more apparent, and it is, unquestionably, an important factor to be taken into consideration in connection with the economical production of pork.

So much is this the case that we can safely say, that no farmer is prepared to raise hogs in any considerable numbers, unless provided with pasture and grass lands, in which abundant water and shade are accessible at all times; with such, hogs will thrive and grow, with but little or no grain, from early spring until the new crop of corn is fit for use, and the process of fattening should begin.

This liberty of pasture, affords the growing animals that exercise necessary to health and proper development, and the succulent grasses, rich in muscle and bone-forming materials, are loosening and cooling to the system, tend to keep it free from disease, and counteract the heating and feverish properties of corn. A very important consideration in favor of grass and forage for swine in summer, is its comparatively small cost; as compared with grain-feeding, the expense is merely nominal.

The loss that occurs every year to farmers, from their not realizing and acting upon the fact that the hog is, in in his normal condition, a grass-eating animal, is simply enormous, and it is well settled in the minds of all who have carefully studied the subject, that to keep swine wholly upon the more concentrated and heating foods, is as unnatural and unprofitable as it would be to keep horses or cows in the same manner.

A very interesting experiment in feeding some pigs, and one which illustrates this point, was recently made by the editor of the *National Live Stock Journal.* From a desire to satisfy himself as to whether a portion of grass, or fibrous food, fed in connection with corn meal, was not more healthful and profitable than the meal without other admixture, he made the experiment of which he thus speaks :

"Taking a litter of six pigs, five weeks old, we divided them into two lots, as nearly equal in weight and thrift as could be done with the eye. This was on the 1st of June. One lot of three was put into a pen, and fed upon corn meal soaked in water twelve hours, *ad libitum.* The other lot was put into a pen alongside, and fed upon green clover, cut short by a straw-cutter, and mixed with corn meal. At first only one quart of this cut clover was fed each pig, with all the meal they would eat. This meal, being mixed with clover, the particles were separated, and when eaten, went into the stomach in a spongy condition, so that the gastric juice could penetrate the mass as water a sponge. The gastric juice came in contact with every part of the mass at once, and the digestion was soon accomplished. This lot of pigs, with the clover and meal, were always lively, always ready for their feed; whilst the other lot, with meal alone, ate greedily for a time, then became mincing and dainty for a few days, showing a feverish state of the system, contenting themselves for a few meals with water, and by fasting got over it, and went on eating again. This was repeated many times during the five months that the experiment lasted. At the end of the time the two lots were weighed. The lot fed on meal alone, weighed 150 lbs. each; the other lot, 210 lbs. each, or 40 per cent. more for being treated as grass-eating animals. Each lot consumed the same amount of meal. The clover, in this case, was given in small quantity, and intended merely to furnish a divisor for the meal. The amount never exceeded two quarts of cut clover at a feed. We have since fed pigs this way, in summer, giving all the cut clover they would eat. This will be found the best way to feed pigs where it is inconvenient to give them a run in pasture. They have always been healthy under this treatment, which we call the normal ration—grass alone, or grass and grain mixed. But larger growth will be made by feeding a small portion of oil meal, mingled with the corn meal and grass; the oil meal being rich in nitrogen and phosphate of lime, to grow the muscle and bone, giving a larger growth to the frame, and thus making more pounds of pork in a given time.

"In order further to test this matter of feeding fibrous food with grain, we experimented, in winter, with two lots of pigs, two in each lot. Each lot weighed 150 lbs. at commencement of experiment, and were all of the same age. The trial continued one hundred and twenty days. One lot was fed corn meal, wet up with hot water, and allowed to stand for a few hours. The other lot was fed a little short-cut clover hay and corn meal, wet up with hot water and allowed to stand. In this case, also, each lot consumed about the same quantity of corn meal. The pigs on meal alone were healthier than those in the other experiments, as they were older, and the weather being cold, were not so feverish. This lot gained 110 lbs. per head, and the lot on clover hay and meal gained 143 lbs. each, or 30 per cent more.

"There is, no doubt, a great loss every year, to the farmers, for not treating the pig as a grass-eating animal, and giving him his normal ration."

It seems to be an unquestionable fact, that the reason why many fail to realize what they might from their swine herds, is that they devote their time and attention almost entirely to the corn field, and utterly ignore the necessity for, or value of, pasture and green food in the summer season. In their eagerness to secure an abundance of winter and fattening food, they fail to encourage rapid growth upon healthful and inexpensive food in the most favorable months of the year.

Various estimates and tables have been prepared by scientific men, to show the amount of nutritive material an acre of land will produce, in cereals and grass, and a fair average of their conclusions on the subject is shown in the following table: The estimate of the product of an acre of clover is quite low, as, when well matured, an acre can, in a favorable season, be made to yield more than the amount here given. The table is on the basis that four pounds of the raw material will make one pound of pork, except that for clover, fifteen pounds is allowed for a pound of pork.

	Gross Product per acre.		*Pork per acre.*	*Value, at 4 cts. per lb.*
	No. bush.	*lbs.*	*lbs.*	
Wheat	15	900	225	$9.00
Barley	35	1,680	420	16.80
Oats	40	1,320	320	13.20
Corn	40	2,240	560	22.40
Peas	25	1,500	375	15.00
Green clover	6 tons	12,000	800	32.00

If this is true in practice, it is evident that an acre of clover is worth, for pork-making, as much as 3 1/2 acres of average wheat, almost as much as 1 1/2 acre of good corn, and nearly as much as 2 1/2 acres of good oats. Hogs that have made most of their growth on corn, have stomachs too small to be the most successful grass-feeders, or make large gains on bulky food of any sort. Swine that are expected to make the most gain on a grass diet, should previously be allowed a portion of food sufficiently bulky to properly distend their stomachs, without which they will lack *carrying room.*

Hog pastures, in July and August, if the weather is quite dry, are likely to become short of forage, and much of the ground rooted over; in this case the stock must have extra attention. Provision can be made for such emergencies by sowing a crop of peas at the proper season, and for swine in warm weather, there are few kinds of food equal to peas. Two bushels, sown broadcast on an acre of properly-prepared land, should produce about thirty bushels of shelled peas, which the hogs will harvest, and if not too ripe, peas, pods, vines, and all, will be eaten.

The value of the field pea is not known or appreciated by the western farmers as it should be, and as it is likely will be, in the future; they produce more flesh in proportion to fat than corn, and are fit for use at a season when especially needed. In England, where it is impossible to raise corn, farmers rely largely on peas to fatten their pork; while in Canada, where very fair corn is raised, they claim that more hog food can be provided from an acre of peas than from an acre of corn.

We are of the opinion that the time is near at hand, when an important food for swine is to be furished in the Jerusalem Artichoke; sometimes called the Brazilian Artichoke, an incorrect name, as the plant is not known in Brazil. While but little information has been given to the public as to the best variety, or manner of producing them, they are held in high estimation by those who have given them a fair trial.

Mr. A. C. Williams, of Vinton, Iowa, a very prominent and successful breeder of Poland-Chinas, in large numbers, says:

"The keep of my hogs, in warm weather, is Blue grass, Clover, and Brazilian Artichokes. Forty head of hogs, and their pigs, may be kept without other food on an acre of Artichokes, from the time frost is out of the ground until the first of June, and from September, or October, until the ground is again frozen.

"To grow them, the ground should be rich, plowed eight or ten inches deep, the tubers cut same as seed potatoes, and planted from early spring to June 10th, ten to fifteen inches apart, in rows that are three feet apart, with six bushels of seed to the acre.

"They can also be planted in the fall, from October 15th to November 15th, but the tubers should not be cut, and the ground should be throughly rolled after planting.

"If planted in spring, plenty of rain in July and August will make them large enough to turn hogs on in September, otherwise not until a month later. If in foul ground, they may, when three or four inches high, be given a thorough working with cultivators, and when the hogs have been removed, to allow a new crop of tubers to grow, the ground should be made smooth by harrowing, that the tops may be cut with a mower, as food for horses and cattle.

"Enough seed will remain in the ground for another crop, but they can easily be eradicated by mowing off the tops and plowing the ground deeply in July and the early part of August.

"The Brazilian Artichoke is red, does not spread and scatter like the wild, white variety, and produces more hog-feed to the acre than any crop I am acquainted with, and the hogs will harvest the crop themselves.

"Hogs taken from the artichoke pastures to clover and blue-grass, will not root up the sod, as they are free from intestinal worms, constipation, indigestion, and fever, caused by feeding corn in winter."

The editor of the *Stock Journal*, writing of Mr. Williams' hogs, as seen at the Iowa State Fair of 1876, said:

"Mr. Williams, of Vinton, had on exhibition one of the largest displays of Poland-Chinas we have ever seen on any fair ground from a single individual. Mr. W. captured the first prize on sows over one year and under six months, and the second on a pair of pigs under six months, in a ring of 28 entries, and a recommended herd premium. Mr. Williams informed us that his herd was taken off his pastures and artichoke fields without any previous fixing up."

Considering how the majority of premium hogs and pigs are pampered and "fixed up" before they are taken to State Fairs, this is a very high compliment to Mr. Williams' "keep." A gentleman writing to the *Prairie Farmer* from Wakarusa, Kansas, speaks of artichokes as follows:

"The Jerusalem Artichoke, in this State, forms a large tuber, (those of over a pound in weight being nothing unusual), is wonderfully productive, very nutritious, and is well liked by the hogs, even in a raw state.

"I planted a few last year to raise seed for this season; and in digging them I found that they had taken entire possession of the ground, so that I had to dig up all the ground between the rows as well as between the hills, and the largest and finest tubers were found deep down in the compact sub-soil where the plow had never reached.

"Here I am reminded of the only objection (so-called) that I have ever heard urged against the artichoke; which is, that if they once get into a piece of ground they never can be eradicated. This, instead of being a valid objection, is really one of the strongest arguments in favor of its use for the purpose under consideration.

"I think that in seeding hog pastures to the artichoke, a division fence should be run through the middle, so that one half could rest each alternate year, and not be disturbed during the growing season. Enough, in any event, would be left in the ground for seed, but in this way the tubers would have a better chance to mature.

"In selecting a piece of ground for hog pasture, (if intended to be planted with artichokes), it will be best to take a rich, moist soil, though they will grow in any soil that is suitable for potatoes. Having made the selection with due care and forethought, let that piece be dedicated forever to the artichoke, when it will be seen that the impossibility of its eradication becomes its highest recommendation, for no further labor will ever be required in planting, cultivating, or digging; the swine will have plenty of the best of summer food, *and they will cultivate it and dig it themselves.*"

The following, to the same journal, was from an Illinois correspondent:

"I have raised the Jerusalem Artichoke on my place twelve years. Soil the same as the common prairies of Iowa and Illinois, and my experience proves them to be a very valuable and useful crop. All kinds of stock, horses, cattle, sheep, and hogs, and chickens, are fond of them. I regard them as very healthy food, and necessary in addition to grain, in the spring, and at this time, are feeding them to my milch cows with the best results.

"One can commence using them in September, and from thence to June, but to use them when the ground is frozen solid, they must be gathered and heaped, and covered with straw and earth, otherwise, whenever the ground can be got into they can be used; being frozen in the ground tends to make them crisp and sweet. Plenty of artichokes and a little corn brings the hogs out fine in the spring, and they will dig them themselves, and will do the same in the fall.

"I was warned by my neighbors, when I got them, to look out or they would get my farm, and take my place to its ruin, but this has not been my experience. I always consoled myself that if they got the advantage of me and grew spontaneously, the struggle would be between them and weeds, the difference being, the artichokes would have roots at the bottom, and the weeds nothing. The only difficulty has been to keep a sufficiency of roots beyond the reach of hogs, to renew my crop with. Cultivate same as potatoes, and same amount of seed, will yield five to one of potatoes, with same culture, and are much easier to cultivate, as they have a strong upright stalk. Plant in the spring; any time in April will do best; I would plant in May rather than miss. Soil cannot be too rich."

The following also appeared in the *Burlington* (Iowa) *Hawkeye*, about the same time:

"Last spring I planted a double handful of small tubers, cut still smaller, I think about 40 pieces, and about 35 plants grew in two rows about 35 feet long (11 steps). A few days ago I dug them, and they were over seven bushels. I threw over the last dug bushel to the pigs and they eat them with avidity. I knocked the dirt off a large one, and offered it to the horse at the garden fence, and he eat it. Three of the best plants yielded each one-half bushel even full, and the majority yielded over a peck each. They were planted in good, moist ground, and hoed once. The six bushels are now in a heap in my garden, and I intend to plant most of them. In spading up where my garden fence had been, I found those tubers in the ground. They were there 18 years ago, when we came here, and how much longer, probably the former owner could tell. One of your correspondents is wrong about the artichoke being impossible to eradicate. I once planted some, and in the autumn turned in hogs, (without knowing anything about the field), and the next spring inclosed it in a calf pasture, and the following spring none appeared. The yield per acre would certainly be enormous, and freezing does no injury. This saves much labor of digging before frost, or digging at all for hogs."

The common method of feeding corn, alone, twelve months in the year, is favorable to the production of the well-known "land pikes," so common on the farms of the West, a few years since, and tens of thousands of hogs have been lost by the so-called "hog cholera," and other diseases, wholly and directly the result of defective and unnatural feeding. We look upon more and better grass, shade, and water, with less dry corn, fed in mud, filth, and dust, as the great panaceas for the many ailments with which such enormous numbers of hogs are annually afflicted and lost. A practical and well known western writer was not far from the facts, when he said, in 1872:

"With many of those who raise hogs in the West, but little attention is paid to their natures, habits, wants, or feed lots; the latter are allowed to become a noisome pestilence, and the only wonder is that the whole race of swine is not exterminated by cholera, blind-staggers, etc., engendered by these sink-holes of iniquity."

In a series of carefully prepared articles written for the *Prairie Farmer*, by Hon. Elmer Baldwin, of Illinois, he makes the following fair statements about the desirability of pasture and forage for swine:

"The farmer who proposes to make money by raising pork, must have a pasture for his swine during the season of grass. Without it the balance is very apt to be on the wrong side of the ledger after selling his crop.

"Clover is supposed to be the best, but Timothy is doubtless equally good. Swine like it about as well, and it is more nutritious. Blue-grass does well, when better is not to be had; even a field of weeds is better than no pasture, as many varieties of weeds are excellent feed. Many a poor widow has made a good porker almost solely on weeds from her garden.

"Where a sufficient range of pasture cannot be had, soiling does well. Clover or Timothy cut when green and fresh, and fed regularly, is the next best feed to a good range of pasture.

"As soon as the grass starts in the spring, the hogs should be turned in, as they like it best when short and tender. They will subsist and grow well on grass alone, with a little salt occasionally. Some prefer to feed a little corn daily; it may or may not be good policy; they will be farther advanced for fattening, but will not fatten as well as if none is fed in summer, and with good pasture, water, and shade, they will give satisfactory results. They will not fatten on grass, but it prepares them for fattening.

"Their systems are in a healthy state. They have no ulcerated livers and stomachs, as they will have if fed on corn through the hot weather.

"Thus kept, they are prepared by the first of September to commence the fattening process, with sound teeth, good digestion, and vigorous health. They will after that time promptly pay for all the feed judiciously given. It may be, and doubtless is, true, that a light feed of bran or light provender might be fed with profit during the summer; but it is doubtful if corn in any quantity is beneficial.

"Feeding on corn alone, during the summer, except it to be send them to a summer market, is bad policy; they become unhealthy, teeth sore, appetites cloyed, and they will not feed satisfactorily in the fall, and the comparative expense of grass and corn feeding must be drawn as to which is the best policy. The cost of grass feeding, even with other light feed, is merely nominal, while a hog fed on corn, from the time it is weaned from the sow until butchered at eighteen months old, can seldom pay expenses.

"The chief end of a hog is the weight and quality of his carcass. His value depends upon his being well fattened, and the object aimed at during his whole life is to prepare him for that event. If he fails in that, his life is a failure.

"Corn is the proper food for fattening, but not for growth; and the fattening process is always, to some extent, a disease-producing process, and if too long continued is always so.

"But when the animal commences fattening in vigorous health, having lived for months on green vegetable and light food, his health will remain firm through any reasonable time required to become fat. But if fed uninterruptedly on heavy, hearty, dry food for all his life, his health, if not already destroyed, is injured, and will yield to such unnatural living before there is time to fatten, as will be shown by loss of appetite, restlessness, unnatural craving for lime, clay, bones, hen-dung, etc. A hog thus affected can not be fattened more that season; he had better be slaughtered, (although it is doubtful if his carcass is fit for food), or turned out for a year, to recuperate.

"It is a common practice to endeavor to counteract this tendency to disease by feeding sulphur, coal, bones, clay, rotten wood, etc., which may be, to some extent, beneficial; but it is like the drugs used to infuse life and health into the gouty, rheumatic, apoplectic, epicurean biped. The health thus obtained is of an inappreciable amount compared with that of the hardy rustic who never had gout or apoplexy. The hog is an epicurean philosopher; and as Providence deals with his biped prototype, (the votary of that philosophy), by throwing in disease at the proper time to close the scene, so the butcher's knife should do for the quadruped what Providence does for the biped, but a little in advance, just before the disease is developed. That is, the fattening process should be completed as soon as possible, (and before disease supervenes), both for economy, and to insure a good, healthful quality of meat, and when the proper amount of fat is laid on, the animal should be slaughtered at once."

It must appear to any candid observing man that the use of grasses, peas, artichokes, etc., instead of corn, for the summer diet of hogs, must be rational and profitable, in producing healthier animals, affording a fairer remuneration to the raiser, and, above all, food more nearly fit for the human stomach.

PASTURE; let this word be written in capitals, by every man who raises swine—*it is the secret of success.*

CHAPTER XIV.

FATTENING.

Healthy swine, of good breed, that have been previously kept in such a manner, and for such a length of time, (the latter depending largely on the breed) as to develop a good-sized and properly formed frame, if put upon full, but not too concentrated, feed in the early days of September, are expected to, and will, lay on flesh very rapidly. The quantity will vary, with different animals, from half a pound to two and a half pounds per day, the latter quantity, however, being quite extraordinary.

Whatever the season of the year, or the number of animals to be fattened, it is important that the enclosure in which they are kept and fed, should have good surface drainage; if possible, there should be plenty of running water, that their feed-lots may not become miry, and to prevent the necessity of the animals drinking from impure sloughs, or mud-holes.

With the best management, it is not desirable that more than about forty head should be confined to less than an acre of ground; though it is frequently the practice to feed that, or a greater number, in a much smaller space, where they are compelled to eat, drink, and sleep in their own filth; after some months of this treatment, if not carried off by that ever convenient scapegoat, "cholera," they become a good and fair quality of—*carrion*. If any considerable number are to be fattened, and the large, medium, and small-sized hogs can be fed by themselves, in different pens or lots, it is an excellent plan to do this; and if not more than fifteen, twenty, or twenty-five are kept together, they will be more peaceable, feed better, gain faster, and be healthier, than if huddled together indiscriminately, to spend their time in continual turmoil and uproar. To be more precise about the space fattening hogs should have, we consider any space sufficient in which a reasonable number are afforded comfort, cleanliness, and a moderate degree of exercise; while any pen is too small, that compels any number to be filthy and uncomfortable.

When taken from grass, or other bulky diet, to be fattened, the change to a more concentrated food should be gradual, as too sudden a change is sometimes attended with injurious effects, if not the loss of some animals outright. They should, at first, have light feed. Bran and other mill-stuff, made into slop, and given with their grain, is good, and if the refuse from the orchard and potato field is given them, it will be beneficial, and especially so, if cooked and mixed with bran, meal, etc.

Our own custom is, to plant early in the spring a piece of good, rich ground, with some of the larger kinds of sweet corn, or an early variety of field corn, and with it put some pumpkin seeds in every sixth or eighth hill, each way. Early in the season this corn is in "roasting-ear," when we begin feeding it to the hogs, stalk and all—as much as they will clean up. It seems exactly suited to their appetites, and starts them along in growth and fattening in a manner that is always gratifying. Cutting the early corn from the ground hastens the growth of the pumpkins, which then begin ripening, and are soon fit for use.

After the hogs have eaten every mouthful of the green corn that they will, we give them as many pumpkins as they want, and usually, each grown hog will eat one good-sized pumpkin, or more. Before they are given to the hogs, the pumpkins should be chopped open, and all, or most all, of the seeds removed, as in large quantities they affect the urinary organs very injuriously, and so derange an animal's system as to make him nearly worthless for any purpose.

We consider that the pork made in this way, at this time of year, yields us as much clear profit as any we produce. We like to cut up corn for the hogs as late in the season as they will eat a good portion of the fodder, and after this, it requires but a few weeks of feeding on clear corn to fully ripen them for slaughter. We differ from many experienced feeders, in believing that the new corn will fatten hogs faster than that a year or two old; but for finishing off a lot of porkers for market, we readily concede that a plenty of old sound corn is good enough for anybody.

As to continuing the use of pumpkins, we never succeeded in raising too many, or in keeping them into the winter longer than we liked to feed them, but fattening hogs should fill up with a full meal of corn before being given the pumpkins, else they would eat too much pumpkin in proportion to the corn, and be very slow in storing up fat. Pumpkins, like wheat bran, are useful adjuncts to the more concentrated kinds of food, but alone cannot be depended on for fattening purposes.

If there is soft, or poor corn to be fed out, it should be used first, as, after beginning to feed, a change from strong, sound feed, to that which is poor and chaffy, is usually for the worse. Any change during the feeding season should be from light to heavier, and more nutritious food, and never the reverse. When, by gradually increasing the quantity of fattening food, the hogs have become accustomed to it, they should be given at regular hours, early in the morning, at noon, and late in the evening, as much corn as they will eat up clean, but no more.

This caution is applicable to all other foods as well as corn, though we are aware that comparatively few hogs are fattened in the corn-growing regions, except upon corn in the ear, and probably the time is far off when it will be otherwise.

So easily and abundantly raised, it has become the principal food for fatting all kinds of farm stock, and being so common, is fed in many cases without a proper knowledge of its adaptability to the animal economy, as is shown by the constant tendency to disease and degeneracy in our domestic animals. Its exclusive use is not the best economy, but being so easily produced, and in such convenient form for feeding, especially in cold weather, it is simply courting ridicule to protest against it; we will, nevertheless, venture to introduce here an item embodying the views endorsed by many of the most learned scientists; it is from the report (see Ch. XXIV.), made in the fall of 1876, to the Missouri State Board of Agriculture, by Dr. Detmers, V. S. This gentleman was commissioned by the Board to investigate the so-called "Hog Cholera," in its various forms and phases, its symptoms and causes, and to suggest means of prevention, and rational treatment.

He writes as follows:

"Finally, I wish to say a few words in regard to a hygienic mistake committed on almost every farm in the west. I refer to the practice of feeding the swine exclusively with corn, a practice which certainly is not calculated to produce healthy and vigorous animals, but which necessarily must result, as I shall try to show, in weakening the organism, and in creating a predisposition to disease. How much or how little this practice has contributed in producing the now prevailing epizootic influenza of swine I am not prepared to decide. I have, however, reasons to suppose that this practice has not been without influence. The organism of a domestic animal is composed of about fifteen to twenty elements, or undecomposable constituents of matter, united in numerous organic compounds. A constant change of matter is taking place, and a part of these elements, in form of organic compounds, is constantly wasted, and carried off by the processes of secretion and excretion. The organism, therefore, in order to remain healthy, and to maintain its normal composition, must receive, from time to time, an adequate supply of those elements, contained in suitable or digestible organic compounds, so as to cover the continual loss, and, if the animal is young, to produce growth and development. The simplest way to introduce these elements into the animal organism is to give food which contains them in nearly the right proportions. A few of these elements, besides hydrogen and oxygen, are sometimes in the form of suitable compounds in limited, though very seldom sufficient, quantities in the water for drinking; for instance, calcium, in the form of lime, iron, etc. One important element—oxygen—enters the organism, also, in large quantities, through the lungs and through the skin, but all others have to be introduced wholly, or almost wholly, in the form of food. Almost all kinds of food, however, milk perhaps excepted, lack some important elements in their composition, contain others in insufficient quantities, and still others in greater abundance than required. Therefore, if such a kind of food is given exclusively—corn, for instance—which is destitute of some of the mineral elements, and contains only an insufficient quantity of nitrogenous compounds, which are of so great importance in the animal organization, irregularities and disorders, in the exercise of the various functions and organs, will be the unavoidable results."

Prof. S. A. Knapp, an extensive breeder of thoroughbred swine, at Vinton, Iowa, to satisfy himself that too much corn, without other food, was detrimental to the health of pigs, made some experiments, one of which he speaks of as follows:

"Two years since, I experimented in feeding dry corn and water to a thrifty, vigorous pig, about twelve weeks old. In three weeks there were indications of fever; the fourth week he became stiff in his limbs, extremely costive, with skin dry—appetite yet good. The fifth week there was great weakness in the hind parts—swelling of the sheath, retention of urine, costiveness, and fickle appetite. The diet was then changed to dish-water and cooked bran drinks; in three weeks the pig was apparently well."

If kept in dry lots, or fed in pens, plenty of trough room should be provided, and at least twice a day the hogs should have as much clean water as they will drink, and practical men know that this is no inconsiderable quantity.

Whatever the feed may be, it should be given in such a manner that they will be forced to eat as little filth as possible, and if corn can be fed on a clean floor, or ground having a sod, it is an excellent plan. But when the animals, to get their feed, must swallow as much mud and manure as grain, but poor results can be expected.

Regularity, as to times of feeding, and quality and quantity of feed, should be observed; no animal should be fed so as to become surfeited, and only so much food should be given at once as will be entirely consumed, that all may come to the next meal with sharp appetites. The most perfect development does not depend so much upon the large quantity they can be made to consume, as upon the quantity they properly digest and assimilate. Next to good food for the appetite, a good appetite for the food is desirable, and should be carefully promoted; the hog that refuses to eat, even for a single day, is set back in his fattening for two or three days, and sometimes for a fortnight. In fact, the failure of a hog's appetite denotes something radically wrong with him, if not with the entire herd and its management. The quantity of food will vary somewhat, and usually in frosty or freezing weather, more will be eaten, to maintain the animal heat, than when the temperature is higher and the atmosphere contains considerable moisture. Good feeding consists in giving every particle the hogs will eat, without leaving any, or losing their appetites, and to accomplish this, intelligent care and close observation are necessary. The old saying, that the lazy farmer, who sits on the fence watching his hogs until they are through eating, generally markets the heaviest pork, is in exemplification of the rules of proper care in feeding. Quiet and comfort are indispensable to thrift, so dogs and boisterous boys should be kept away from the feed lots and pens. We have always found it convenient to accustom our hogs to some particular call, which will bring them together, and sometimes they can thus be called into places where it would be about impossible to drive them.

We salt our own hogs, by putting small quantities in their swill, and sulphur is given in the same way. Bituminous or soft coal, charcoal, wood ashes, and rotten wood, are relished by hogs as condiments, and we think that these should be kept within their reach.

Comfortable, sheltered beds, not too deep and dusty, are equivalent to a considerable amount of food, as stock suffering from cold cannot thrive, and to warm them with grain, applied internally, is much more expensive than good nests and shelter, applied externally.

One hundred pounds of pork from ten bushels of corn, is the usual estimate made by western farmers who feed whole corn, but fed in a different form, and in conjunction with other food, it will make much more, as has been many times fully demonstrated by careful feeders, both in America and Europe. The example of the farmers in the New England States is valuable, as they are noted for raising the best of pork with small corn crops, and no "cholera." The general method pursued

"Is to commence fattening by boiling potatoes, pumpkins, apples, or other vegetables, and mix a little bran, shorts, or provender, with the cooked vegetables when hot, thus thoroughly cooking the meal. It is theh placed in tubs or vats, and allowed to slightly ferment, when it is ready for use. The amount of meal is gradually increased until near killing time, when meal well cooked is given alone.

"The meal is composed of oats, buckwheat, and corn, or any other coarse grain, or of any two of them, generally finishing with corn meal alone. Thus treated, they fatten much faster than on dry corn, and at much less expense. It costs more labor, but at a season when it can be well spared, and it is well recompensed.

"The English system is still more diversified. They use all kinds of vegetables—potatoes, turnips, carrots, beets, peas, beans, barley, and oats; the grain steamed or ground; the vegetables cooked and mixed with slop from the house, dairy, distillery, brewery, etc. Even grass and clover is cut and mixed with the feed, and almost every substance of light cost and any nutriment, is nicely prepared and finds a ready market in the maw of the omnivorous hog."

We do not wish to be understood as arguing, in this chapter, or in this book, that corn is not a suitable food for swine, or that it is not the *best* single fat-producing material for the money in the world, for general use ; but would enforce the fact that a variety is essential to perfect health and development in *all* animals, and a single article of food becomes satisfactory to none,—not even to a hog.

A very satisfactory method of fattening hogs, largely

practised in the west by those who "stall feed" cattle, is to put shotes, of one hundred to one hundred and fifty pounds weight, with the cattle whenever grain feeding is begun—generally about the first of October—at the rate of fifteen to twenty shotes to ten steers, the number depending on the amount of grain used, and the manner in which it is placed before the cattle. In the fine weather of fall and early winter, it is common to feed corn in the fodder, or in the shuck, by throwing it upon the grass in the pasture; the favorite way is to feed in two different enclosures, and each day to turn the hogs into the one where the cattle were fed the day previous; this enables them to pick up the leavings of the cattle, without trampling on and over the day's feed, until the cattle have eaten as much of it as they wish.

When full feed is given to cattle in this way, about two shotes to each steer is not too many, but when corn is fed in tight boxes and troughs, so that but a small proportion is scattered, from one shote to one and a half per steer will keep the feed lots well gleaned.

If a greater number are kept, they will need to have extra grain given them, in order to fatten rapidly; but if simply growth is the object, three shotes will fare pretty well in following each steer that is on full feed.

The grain voided whole by the cattle seems to be so softened and so digestible, that hogs thrive on it amazingly, so that the larger ones are soon in a condition for market, and others can occupy their places in the feeding lots.

Hogs seldom fatten more satisfactorily, rapidly, or with less outlay of labor, than when handled in this way, and the plan is justly held in high favor, from the fact that every pound of increase from the droppings and scattered corn is clear gain, none of which could be utilized without the much-abused hog.

One common defect in this method of managing hogs

is, that they are not generally provided with suitable sleeping quarters, where they can be comfortable, without crowding, and out of danger of being trampled and horned by the cattle.

Autumn, with its mild weather, is the profitable season for making pork and lard, and hogs not fed with cattle, should be far along in their fattening before severe winter weather sets in. When hogs become so fat as to get up and about with difficulty, it is a loss to feed them longer, and the packer and the barrel should take them in.

In feeding soft or cooked food, a kerosene barrel mounted on wheels will answer, but where something not quite so high, and less circumscribed at the top can be constructed, it will be found more convenient.

CHAPTER XV.

COOKING FOOD FOR SWINE.—FOOD COOKERS.

The question as to the economy and general desirability of cooking food for swine, has long been a subject of discussion and speculation, yet there probably is quite as much diversity of opinion, among farmers in general at the present day, as at any previous time.

The surrounding conditions and circumstances, have much to do in deciding the question of economy; and while one farmer, under certain circumstances, could feed a considerable portion of cooked grain and secure satisfactory returns therefor, another, differently situated, though perhaps in the same neighborhood, and raising the same class of swine, might be unable to do so without actual loss.

Under favorable circumstances many have, by careful experiments, thoroughly satisfied themselves that the practice of cooking is largely profitable, and others, from experiments fully as careful and thorough, have arrived at conclusions directly the reverse.

There can scarcely be a doubt that cooking hard, dry corn, renders it more easy of digestion, enabling the animal to extract the maximum of nutritive material it contains, and that, ordinarily, fed in this form and of the proper consistency, it affords a larger percentage of flesh and fat, than if fed in the raw state. A large majority, we think, of those who have given attention to the subject, admit this; at the same time, a respectable and intelligent minority, vote *nay.* That it is practically profitable, on a majority of farms, to pursue a system of cooking the food for large stocks of swine, is not generally conceded.

Among the reasons for regarding cooking as impracticable, are, the scarcity of timber for fuel, the extra labor involved, and the general lack of fixtures and facilities for cooking, and feeding the food in its cooked state.

Vast numbers of those whose farms are located in the best corn-growing regions, would, by the single item of fuel, be deterred from undertaking it, even if convinced that cooking would give, from the cooked food, a considerable increase of flesh and fat over that consumed raw.

Others, with fuel convenient and abundant, and fully satisfied of the importance and economy of feeding cooked grain, are practically prevented from carrying out their convictions, by the scarcity and expense of reliable, intelligent help. There are others still, with so much wood and timber, that it is a burden, and who have help to spare, yet having no very decided views for or against cooking, suppose that some hundreds of dollars would have to be expended in buying, fitting up, and learning to use the very simplest apparatus that would possibly answer. We shall try to disabuse the minds of this last mentioned classs further on in this chapter.

The Messrs. H. M. & W. P. Sisson, of Galesburg, Illinois, in a pre-eminently prairie country, are uncommonly successful breeders of swine in large numbers, and, at some seasons of the year, use a considerable quantity of cooked food. Knowing them to be practical men, pursuing their business for profit, rather than for the purpose of demonstrating any preconceived theories, we solicited of them a statement of their conclusions, from experience, as to the profit and desirability of cooking food for swine, on a small, medium, and large scale. In their reply, they express views so nearly identical with those entertained by us, that we cheerfully present their conclusions in lieu of our own. They write:

"We have been cooking food for hogs, more or less, for the last six or eight years, and we state as the result of our experience and observation, that in the great hog and corn producing States, cooking food for hogs, *generally*, will not pay; still, there are times and circumstances which will make cooking, to a limited extent, profitable.

"We do not think it profitable to cook corn, or meal, for hogs, whenever they can have access to good, tender grass, and the temperature is such that corn can be soaked in water. Soaking will then answer every purpose, but in winter, when there is no grass, and dry corn is the principal food, is the time that cooking will pay, if ever.

"Hogs need something besides dry corn, (it is too concentrated), something with more bulk; and to meet this requirement, we do some cooking. If a slop is made of corn and oat meal, middlings and bran, and finished up with potatoes, pumpkins, or squashes, all well cooked, and fed in connection with dry corn, we think the advantage will be very apparent.

"It is not absolutely necessary that this should be fed more than once a day, but *pigs*, especially, should have enough, once a day, to fill up and properly distend the stomach. In speaking of pigs, we mean those six months old, or more.

"It is our opinion, that the disease known as hog cholera, is very largely occasioned by the almost exclusive use of corn. Hogs should have a variety of food; they need something besides corn; oats, bran, potatoes, etc., fed for a change, and for variety, are very beneficial.

"We use a simple pan, or boiler, that has an iron bottom and ends, with plank sides, so that the contents can be drawn off into a vat. The boiler has a light cover, and is about eight feet long, three feet wide, and fifteen inches deep. Such an arrangement is cheap, and can be made profitable, principally in winter.

"We will say, in conclusion, that we do not believe that it will pay, either on a small, medium, or large scale, to generally substitute cooked for uncooked food, for hogs in the great hog and corn-producing regions of the West."

Mr. Thomas Wood, the successful breeder of Chester Whites, mentioned in another chapter, writes us:

"For the last eight or ten years, I have cooked feed for my hogs, and with the steamer that I have fixed up I can make one or two hogsheads of mush at a time. I cook food as a matter of economy, believing that about one-fourth the grain is saved thereby. I generally feed of corn two parts, and oats one part, ground together, and with this I feed considerable whole corn, particularly in the fall before it gets hard and dry. Feed, when cooked, should be allowed to get nearly cold before it is given to the hogs.

"A few days ago, I weighed and put in separate pens, two sows, in every way the same, and of the same litter. No. 1 weighed 292 lbs., and No. 2 weighed 280 lbs. I fed No. 1 for 17 days on unground corn, cooked; she consumed 2 bushels and 21 quarts, and gained 36 lbs. No. 2 I fed the same length of time, on whole corn, raw, of which she consumed 3 bushels and 13 quarts, and gained 30 lbs.

"The summer before the above experiment was made, I fed eight shotes with corn and oats, (one part oats, and two parts corn), ground, and made it into well-cooked mush, and frequently weighed them, in order to see if it would pay to make pork at the then ruling prices of corn (55c.), oats (40c.), and pork (7c.). The result was that the pork paid nearly two prices, for the corn and oats, while the manure paid for the labor."

U. H. Stowe, of Indiana, had four pigs of a litter, which weighed 245 lbs. each, and four of another litter that weighed 170 lbs. each. He took one of each litter, and put in a pen by itself, and the other six in another pen, and gave both an equal chance, allowing both as much good, sound corn as they could eat, for six weeks. The corn fed to the six was thoroughly cooked whole, and that fed to the two was raw, and fed in the usual way.

The hogs on the raw corn gained ten pounds to the bushel, and those fed on the cooked corn gained just fifteen pounds to the bushel consumed.

Prof. Wilkinson, of Baltimore, says: "I conducted an agricultural school and experimental farm for eight years, and experimented with feeding cooked food of every description used for cows, horses, swine, working and fattening cattle, and poultry, and carefully noted the results. These were in all cases very remunerative; so much so, that even with the defective, inconvenient, and expensive apparatus used—for want of better—in steaming, manipulating, and feeding, I found there was an average profit of fully 25 per cent."

THE EXPERIMENTS OF S. H. CLAY.

Readers of agricultural papers have, no doubt, frequently seen allusions to experiments made by Mr. S. H Clay, of Paris, Ky., in cooking food for swine.

Mr. Clay was an extensive breeder of Berkshires, being the gentleman to whom was awarded the grand prize of $1,000, for the finest display of swine at the National Swine Exposition, in Chicago, September, 1871. He made these experiments to settle, in his own mind, the question as to what extent, and under what circumstances, cooking food could be profitably followed.

The experiments were begun July 16th, with six barrows, each about twelve months old, at which time they weighed as follows:

No. 1	255	pounds.
" 2	285	"
" 3	240	"
" 4	240	"
" 5	265	"
" 6	245	"

They were fed together for twelve days on cooked corn meal, reduced to such a consistency that the animals could readily *drink it.* At the end of twelve days, they were separated, when each pig weighed as follows:

No. 1, 294	pounds, having gained	39	pounds.
" 2, 318	" " "	33	"
" 3, 290	" " "	50	"
" 4, 276	" " "	36	"
" 5, 290	" " "	25	"
" 6, 282	" " "	37	"

Nos. 1 and 2 were put in a pen together, and for 30 days fed on boiled corn, consuming 390 pounds, or six bushels and 54 pounds, upon which No. 1 gained 50 pounds, and No. 2 gained 52 pounds, or together, 102 pounds.

For the same period, Nos. 3 and 4 were fed together, in a pen, on meal, boiled and reduced to a thin slop, consuming 254 pounds, or four bushels and 46 pounds, upon which No. 3 gained 30 pounds, and No. 4 gained 50 pounds, or together, 80 pounds.

Nos. 5 and 6 were for the same period fed on dry corn, consuming 405 pounds, or seven bushels and 13 pounds. Upon this, No. 5 gained 10 pounds, and No. 6 gained 32 pounds, or together, 42 pounds.

The following will illustrate the foregoing in tabular form :

	Nos. 1 and 2. Boiled Corn.	*Nos. 3 and 4. Boiled Meal.*	*Nos. 5 and 6. Dry Corn.*
Consumed..................	6 bu. 54 lbs.	4 bu. 46 lbs.	7 bu. 13 lbs.
Gain in 30 days.............	102 lbs.	80 lbs.	42 lbs.
Pork to 1 bushel corn.......	14 $^{65}/_{100}$ lbs.	16 $^{61}/_{100}$ lbs.	5 $^{80}/_{100}$ lbs.
Corn per bushel............	28 cents.	28 cents.	28 cents.
Cost of pork per lb.........	1c. 9 mills.	1c. 6 mills.	4c. 8 mills.

At the end of the 30 days, a change was made, and the hogs fed as follows: Nos. 5 and 6, that had been fed on dry corn, were for the next 26 days given cooked meal; they consumed 234 pounds of meal, equal to 4 bushels and 10 lbs. of shelled corn, upon which No. 5 gained 40 lbs., and No. 6 gained 34 lbs., or together 74 lbs.

Nos. 3 and 4, that had been fed on cooked meal, were fed for the same period of 26 days, on dry corn; they consumed 364 lbs., or 6 $^{1}/_{2}$ bushels, upon which No. 3 gained 34 lbs., and No. 4 gained 10 lbs., or together 44 lbs.

Nos. 1 and 2 were still kept on the diet of boiled corn, with about the same results as in the former trial. The following table shows the results of the 26 days' trial:

	Boiled Meal. Nos. 5 and 6.	*Dry Corn. Nos. 3 and 4.*
Consumed............................	4 bu. 10 lbs.	6 bu. 28 lbs.
Gain in 30 days.......................	74 lbs.	44 lbs.
Pork to 1 bushel corn................	17 $^{72}/_{100}$ lbs.	6 $^{77}/_{100}$ lbs.
Corn per bushel......................	28 cents.	28 cents.
Cost of pork per lb..................	1 cent 5 mills.	4 cents 1 mill.

It appears that, during the twelve days, when the hogs were first put up together and fed cooked meal, No. 5 gained 25 *pounds*, but when they were separated, and fed thirty days on dry corn, the same hog gained but 10 lbs., while it consumed 202 $^{1}/_{2}$ lbs. of corn. With corn at 28 cents per bushel, each pound of pork produced would cost in this case 10 cents and 1 mill; but when in the second trial the hog is again fed on boiled meal, it consumes but 117 lbs. in 26 days, and *gains forty pounds*, and gives the pork gained at a cost of *one cent and four mills per pound.*

In the first period of twelve days, No. 4 made a gain of *thirty-six* pounds, or three pounds per day, on the cooked meal, and being continued on the same food for the thirty days following, consumed but 135 lbs. of meal, and gained thereon *fifty* pounds, at a cost of one cent and three mills for each pound of gain. But the same hog, when fed on dry corn in the second trial, consumed 182 lbs. in *twenty-six* days, and made a gain of only *ten* pounds, at a cost per pound of *nine cents and one mill.*

In his experiment, Mr. Clay obtained from one bushel of corn, fed in the form of cooked meal, about the same quantity of pork that he did from *three* bushels, fed without cooking or grinding. In other words, he found one hundred bushels of dry corn made him less pork than did forty bushels of corn, when ground and cooked. By cooking the feed, he was also enabled to make one hog gain fifty pounds, while another hog, (equal in all respects), gained on dry corn but ten pounds in the same length of time.

That those gentlemen who believe whole or raw corn will make as much or more pork than when cooked, or ground, are not without reasons for the faith that is in them, we are certain, and the following experiments—which we must assume were made as carefully as the others—will not lessen it. The first experiment was made on the farm of the Iowa Agricultural College, by Mr. M. Stalker, the Superintendent, and as some, to whom the results were displeasing, have ridiculed it, and sneered at its author, as a "book farmer," "theorist," and "college professor," it is fair to remark that those who know him, say he is a gentleman pre-eminently distinguished for his strong common sense, with a thorough practical knowledge of the every-day business of farm life.

He reports :

"On the first day of July, (1875), an experiment was commenced, for testing the comparative value of different kinds of food for pigs. The food used was dry corn, soaked corn, cooked corn, dry meal, and cooked meal. Five lots of pigs were selected, as nearly uniform as could be taken from a lot of fifty. Three pigs were put in each pen.

"The pigs were all of Berkshire blood. They were placed in floored pens, and given nothing but their regular allowance of food, with all the water they would drink.

"The corn was all shelled and weighed. During the months of July and August, each lot consumed fifteen bushels of corn, or the same amount ground into meal. The pigs were carefully weighed each week, and a complete record of the results taken.

"During the last week in August, when the weather was extremely warm, pens No. 4 and 5 sustained a small loss, while Nos. 2 and 3 made a slight gain.

"Below are given the results.

	Pen No. 1, fed on dry corn.	Pen No. 2, fed on soaked corn.	Pen No. 3, fed on boiled corn.	Pen No. 4, fed on dry meal.	Pen No. 5, fed on cooked meal.
Weighed July 1	491	520	468	503	519
Weighed September 1	675	660	618	678	676
Gain	184	140	150	175	157
Gain per bushel	12.26	9.33	10.00	11.66	10.46

"On the 1st day of September the pigs were all put upon full feed, each pen receiving the same kind of food as during the first two months.

"The experiment was concluded for each pen when fifteen bushels had been consumed, except No. 2, which had consumed but 13¾ bushels up to October 25th."

	Pen No. 1, fed on dry corn.	Pen No. 2, fed on soaked corn.	Pen No. 3, fed on boiled corn.	Pen No. 4, fed on dry meal.	Pen No. 5, fed on cooked meal.
Weighed September 1	675	660	618	678	676
Weighed October 23	870	......	......	880	......
Weighed October 25	......	800	......	......	818
Weighed October 28	......	.....	780	......	......
Gain	195	140	162	202	142
Gain per bushel	13.00	10.24	10.80	13.46	9.46

"Mr. R. L. Bingham, of Bloomington, Grant county, Wisconsin, states that, after purchasing an Anderson steamer, he commenced, February 15th, an experiment in feeding nineteen pigs, about nineteen weeks old, a cross of Berkshire with common stock. Prior to the experiment, the pigs had the run of the farm, and had been fed as much raw corn as they would eat. Then for a period of twenty-eight days, they were fed as before, with corn in the ear and all the water they could drink. At the close of this period, the total gain in weight was 667 lbs., made from feeding 55 bushels of corn —a gain of 12 lbs. for each bushel of corn. They were then fed with thick mush, made by bringing the water to a boiling heat, and then stirring in the meal ground fine, with the steam still on, allowing the meal to cook five to ten minutes, and adding salt; this was fed to them warm, three times a day, as much as they would eat clean. At the end of twenty-eight days they were again weighed, showing a gain of 676 lbs., made on 75 bushels of corn, less toll—a gain of 9 lbs. for each bushel of corn consumed. He then put 11 of the pigs on raw corn again, continuing to feed the others with cooked meal. May 25, after a trial of six weeks, those on raw corn averaged a gain of 44 lbs. each, and the others an average gain of 37 lbs."

Prof. Henry, of the Wisconsin Experiment Station, has summarized all the most carefully made experiments at educational institutions in America, including those by himself, on a variety of foods, and as a whole they afford a wonderfully strong showing against the practice and profit of cooking for swine. The showing is this:

Agricultural Experiment Station, Wisconsin.	
Cooked barley meal (4 trials) was to uncooked as	93.7 to 100
Cooked corn meal (2 trials) was to uncooked as	81.0 to 100
Cooked corn meal and shorts (2 trials) was to uncooked as	96.1 to 100
Cooked whole corn and shorts (2 trials) was to uncooked as	85.8 to 100
Ontario Agricultural College.	
Cooked peas (2 trials) were to uncooked as	84.9 to 100
Michigan Agricultural College.	
Scalded corn and oatmeal was to wet meal as	101.7 to 100
Kansas Agricultural College.	
Cooked shelled corn was to uncooked corn as	84.0 to 100
Iowa Agricultural College.	
Cooked shelled corn (2 trials) was to uncooked as	82.3 to 100
Cooked corn meal (2 trials) was to uncooked as	79.3 to 100
Maine Agricultural College.	
Cooked corn meal (9 trials) was to uncooked as	82.9 to 100

"It will be noted," observes Prof. Henry, "that in every instance but one, that at the Michigan Agricultural College, there is a loss resulting from cooking; in the exception the gain is very slight, being less than two per cent. Even in this case the meal was not really cooked, but scalded by boiling water being poured on to the meal in a pail and covered up, while the other meal was fed wet with water."

Many other experiments and a vast fund of valuable information have been collated and very lucidly presented in the elaborate article (Chap. XVIII.) prepared by Mr. Joseph Sullivant, of the Ohio State Board of Agriculture. High authority in such matters has said: "No man engaged in pork-raising can afford to pursue his business, without giving Mr. Sullivant's paper careful investigation. He will find there embodied, in a reasonable space, a carefully prepared and full statement of the experiences of many, that it would require him days and perhaps weeks of study and research to obtain."

A FOOD COOKER.

Much money has been wasted in the purchase of various steamers, boilers, cookers, and similar apparatus, patented, high-priced, and highly extolled, at least by patentees, makers, and venders. Not a few credulous persons have been almost persuaded that, if possessed of one of these wonderful inventions, they could raise hogs on so near no grain at all, that a fortune was inevitable, if the business was well followed.

While the apparatus of each different make has some point to recommend it, no great number of meritorious features are combined in any *one* that is simple and cheap, and we have observed that those who invest in this class of merchandise, sooner or later permit it to get out of repair, fall into disuse, and if not left out in the weather, it is stored in some out-building, or corner of the barn, while, in time, the room it occupies is looked upon as being worth more than the old "contraption" itself.

The royalty to the inventor, the manufacturer's profits, the margins to retailers, together with the considerable freights on such heavy wares, make them high in price to the farmers, and the results obtained from them are, in many cases, and from various causes, so unsatisfactory, that the entire experiment is regarded as an expensive failure.

For successful operation, and simplicity and economy in construction, we regard an apparatus made and used

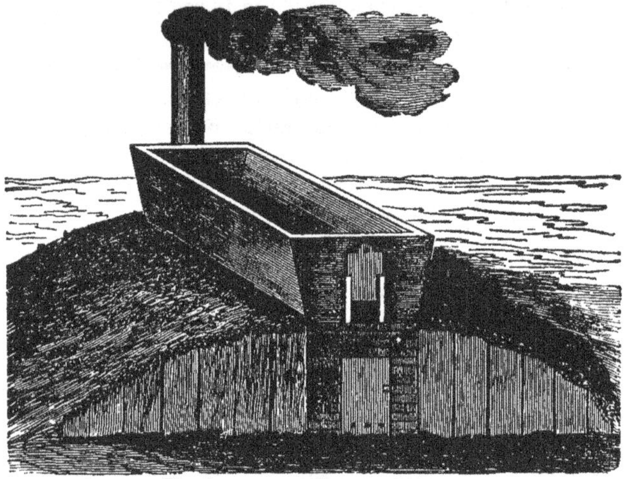

Fig. 7.—MR. CLAY'S FOOD COOKER.

by the late S. H. Clay, of Paris, Ky., as about as good, if not superior to, any patented cooker that could be bought for two or three times the cost of this. It consists of a box two feet wide, and six or eight feet long, and 18 to 24 inches deep, made of two-inch hard-wood plank, and is somewhat wider at the top than at the bottom. The bottom is of heavy sheet iron, nailed firmly to the sides and ends. The box rests on brick or stone walls, high enough to give a plenty of fire-room underneath. A trench in the ground might do in lieu of walls. The front of the fire-place has a door of sheet or cast iron, with a damper, by which to regulate the fire. The door is of sufficient size to permit the use of refuse knots, and the chunks found about the farm or wood-pile.

At the rear end, a chimney, or suitable escape for smoke, is constructed; for this purpose large sized stove-pipe answers well. In making the box, thick white lead should be carefully spread on the bottom edges, before nailing on the iron bottom; this will make it less likely to leak.

After setting the box on the walls, earth is banked up against them; the earth should extend up against the sides of the box somewhat, to prevent the escape of smoke and sparks through the walls.

For drawing off the contents of the box, a sliding gate, with a tin spout under it, is arranged in the front end. A cover, made of inch pine, or other boards, cut on a bevel with the flaring sides of the box, should fit inside of it, instead of on the top, and have some sort of handles at each end for convenience in lifting it.

A few strips of wood, at intervals, on the bottom, and upon them a false bottom, with numerous small perforations, is desirable, as it will prevent meal, or other fine food, from burning at the bottom.

Whenever the box is emptied, it should be cleaned out under the false bottom, and if emptied of food when there is a fire below, some water should be poured in at once, to prevent injury to the pan.

With such an arrangement as this for boiling corn, shelled or in the ear, potatoes, turnips, pumpkins, beets, etc., with cheap fuel, and feeding the mass when cold, or but moderately warm, we believe that almost any farmer can secure a fair compensation for the time and labor expended in cooking a goodly portion of the food for his hogs, and if he cannot do this, surely cooking must be unprofitable.

When it is more suitable to soak the corn than to cook it, the box will be useful for this purpose, and for heating water and scalding hogs, at butchering time, it will indeed be found "a good thing to have in the family."

CHAPTER XVI.

HOG HOUSES AND PENS.

We have seen but few expensive buildings, erected for the use of swine, that were in any great degree satisfactory; the more elaborate and expensive these were, the less desirable and practically valuable they seemed to be.

Large hog houses, usually bring too many animals together, where lack of room, ventilation, and exercise, favor disease and vermin; besides, they increase the difficulty of making suitable arrangements for pasturing, and fail to afford sufficient sunlight, and general comfort.

On most farms, a small or large number of swine can be provided with comfortable housing from such material, and of such construction, as will readily suggest themselves to almost any man fit to be entrusted with the care of stock.

Sleeping apartments should be enclosed on the north-east, and on the west, with a tight wall of stone, boards, logs, or even hay or straw, covered well; in lieu of something better, hay or straw makes a very good roof. The apartments should be open, and front the south, to admit light and warmth from the sun, and should be provided with fresh bedding. Such house will, perhaps, answer as well as one constructed after the elaborate plans of an architect. Reasonable protection from cold and storm, dry, clean bedding, and fresh air are requisite in sleeping apartments for swine, and the farms are few where these cannot be secured at a merely nominal cost.

A well-known western breeder says:

"The common plan of erecting large buildings for the rearing and keeping of swine, is objectionable, upon the ground that, during the season of the year when a pen is particularly required, such buildings are usually cold, dull, and dark, receiving the rays of the sun only a few hours each day.

"Light, air, and sunshine appear to be especially agreeable to the animals, particularly during the fall, winter, and spring months, and are unquestionably conducive to health and growth. Hence, in erecting buildings, or pens, for hogs, these things should be especially looked after, as a cheerful pen will be likely to give you a cheerful pig."

For those desiring a breeding house that is somewhat elaborate, we present the one shown on pages 142 and 143, it having probably had as much careful thought given it, by a practical breeder and farmer, as any similar establishment in the country, and it is not without many useful features to recommend it.

It was planned and erected by a gentleman of practical experience for his farm in Wyandotte County, Kansas.

The building (fig. 8) is 100 feet long by 30 feet wide, built of first quality of pine, upon stone foundations, and arranged with a view to the utmost economy of time and labor in feeding and care of the stock.

By reference to the ground plan (fig. 9), it will be seen that there are fourteen pens on each side. These are divided by movable partitions, so that one or more pens can at any time be thrown together as one. Each pen is furnished with a fender, to prevent the young pigs from being overlaid and smothered by the sow.

Through the centre of the building is a drive-way, 12 feet wide, through which runs a wooden track and truck-car, for carrying barrels of feed from the steamer and feed rooms. Each of the troughs extends through the

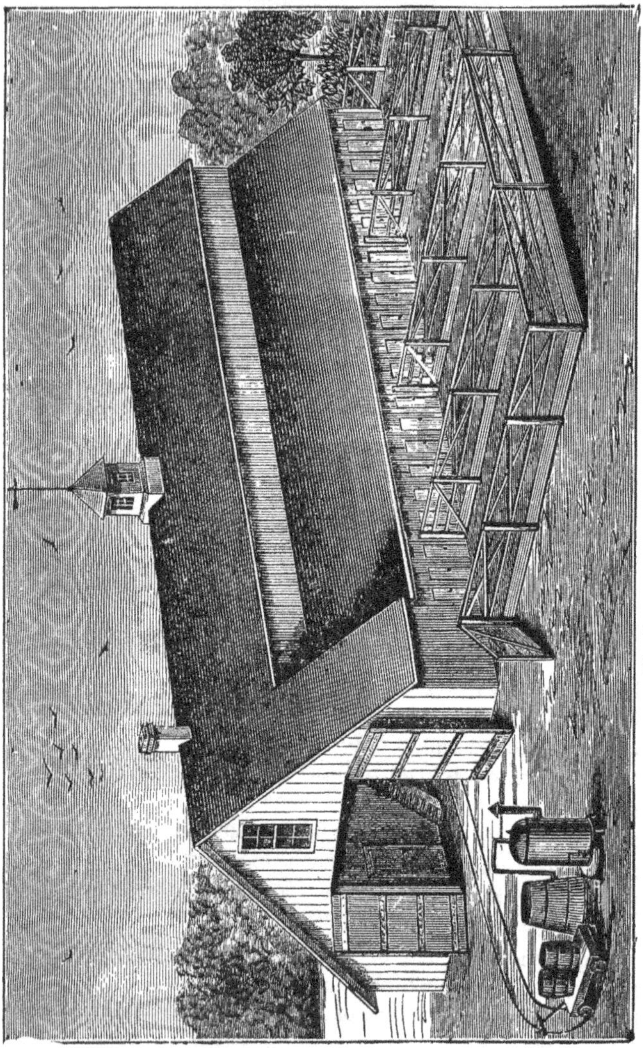

Fig. 8.—VIEW OF A KANSAS PIGGERY.

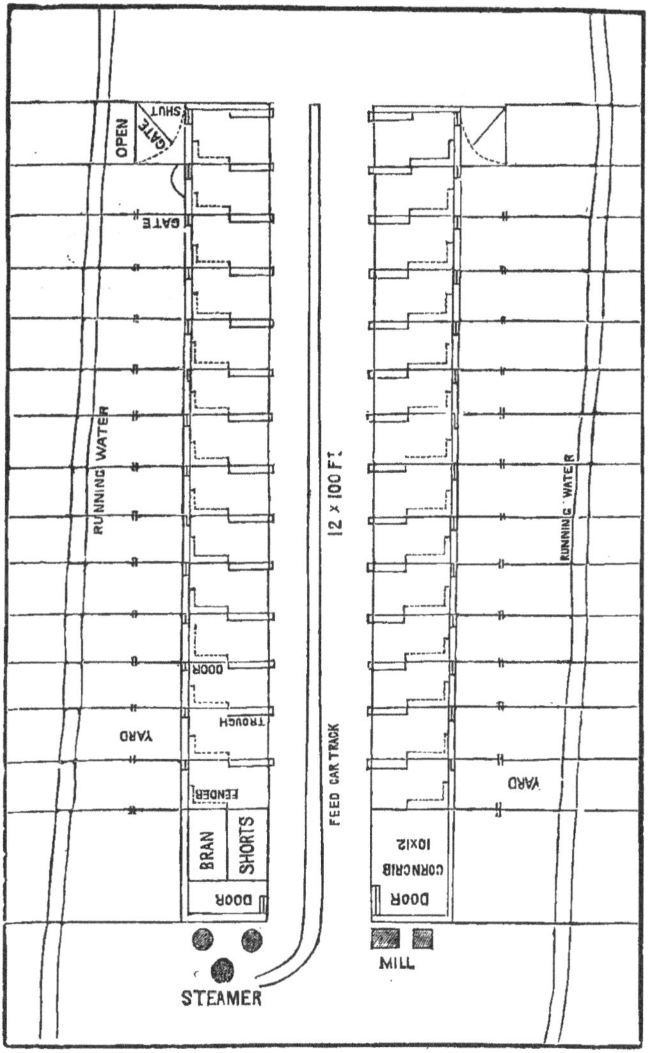

Fig. 9.—PLAN OF THE KANSAS PIGGERY.

partition between the pens and the drive-way, so that feed can be poured into them from the outside, without interference from the animals within.

All of the pens open into outside lots, (it was found impracticable to show them all in the view), the gates between them forming, when open, an alley, through which animals can be readily moved from one portion to another, and manure wheeled out to the compost heap.

Fresh spring water runs through all the out-lots on either side of the building, and extensive clover pastures are accessible from the north, east, and south.

Its owner raised hogs by the hundred, and claims for this establishment that it economizes labor, and affords excellent care and protection to a large number of animals, giving warmth in winter, and shelter and ventilation in summer.

By opening the large doors at each end of the building, and the fourteen small doors on each side, the freest ventilation is secured in both directions; the interior walls of the pens are, of course, but a few feet high, and the space above them open.

In its owner's opinion, the abundant clover pastures adjacent, and the strong, never-failing springs, constantly supplying an abundance of the purest water, are among the chief recommendations of this structure, and they are prime necessities to the success of any other swine-breeding establishment.

Mr. Charles Snoad, Secretary of the National Association of Swine Breeders, contributes to the *Prairie Farmer Annual* the plan of an inexpensive house for swine, a view of which is given in figure 10, and a plan in figure 11. Of this building Mr. Snoad says:

"The plan submitted is one I have just adopted, and, as will be observed, it is so simply constructed, that it can be built by almost any farmer.

"The importance of a southern exposure, for the continued good health and comfort of all animals during the fall, winter, and spring months, will hardly be questioned. In erecting large buildings on the usual plan, these advantages are almost wholly lost sight of. This building is 70 feet in length, and 16 feet in width,

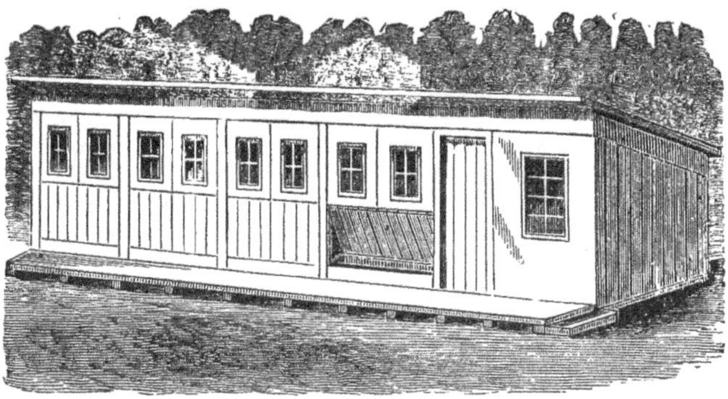

Fig. 10.—VIEW OF MR. SNOAD'S PIGGERY.

including front platform. The cost of it will not exceed $100, with lumber from $17 to $21 per thousand.

"The roof is of stock boards, with a groove cut in each edge, and battened. For cooking or preparing food for the stock, or for the storage of grain, a portion of the building may be appro-

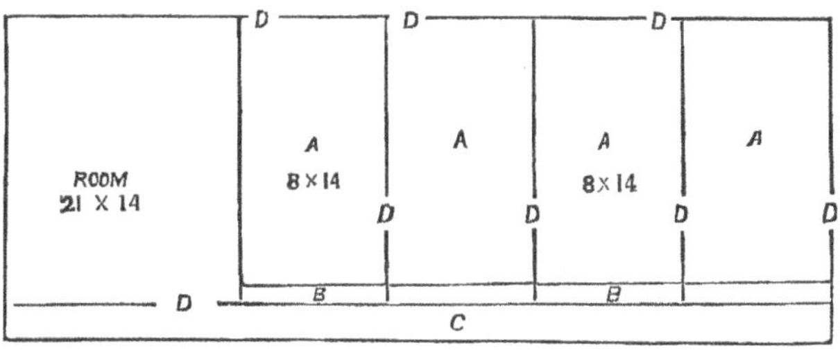

Fig. 11.—PLAN OF MR. SNOAD'S PIGGERY.

(The sash doors are designed to swing in, and the gates to swing back over the troughs, while putting in food.) A, A, Pens, 8×14 feet; B, B, Feed Troughs; C, Platform in front, two feet wide; D, D, D, Doors.

priated, adding to the hight, length, or width, to suit the convenience of the proprietor. Such changes in the division of pens may also be made as may be deemed best.

"The most important features claimed are: warmth, light, air, and sunshine. It may be considered an objection, to be obliged to feed from the outside of the building, but it is believed that the comfort and thrift of the animals, will more than compensate for this apparent additional trouble. Many a cold, cutting day, may be made one of comfort and warmth, by taking advantage of the sunshine.

"In locating the storage and cooking room, the point best adapted to the demands of the case, should be selected. If it is more convenient to do the cooking near the residence, I should have it done there, in preference to using a part of the piggery.

"Many of the steamers or boilers now in use, can be placed in a very small room, and frequently in the dwelling house, conducting the steam to the point desired for cooking the food, through iron gas pipe.

"Modifications and changes are necessary in almost all plans, to adapt them to the wants of different individuals and locations."

An Illinois feeder gives in the *Stock Journal*, Feb., 1877, the plan of a good feeding floor and pen, as follows:

"A floor 30 × 30 feet will give room enough to feed 100 to 120 hogs, and may be made to do twice that service, by feeding a second lot after the first have had time to eat, as I have frequently done for months at a time, and with good satisfaction. The floor should be divided, leaving each part 30 × 15 feet, and each accommodating from 50 to 60 hogs at once, which, I think, is as many as ought to be fed together. The lumber necessary for such floor is about as follows:

3 pieces	6 × 8,	for sills,	30 feet long.......	360 feet.
16 "	2 × 8,	" joists,	16 "	320 "
16 "	2 × 8,	" "	14 "	280 "
1,800 feet	2 × 6,	" floor	....	1,800 "
Common lumber, to enclose (5 feet high)....				600 "
Total....................................				3,360 "

except posts, which may be set upon the sill or into the ground, and will not add materially to the expense—if on the sill, then 28 pieces 4 × 4, 5 feet long, 175 feet, and lumber for division, 100 feet; lumber, all told, 3,635 feet, costing here $13 per thousand, or $47.25 for the whole. The floor might be made of inch lumber, instead of two-inch, as in the bill, but is not so good, nor is it cheaper in the end.

"The sleeping place I prefer, should not be less than 30 or 40 feet from the feed floor, as less manure will be taken there, and it will seldom be wet, as is sure to be the case if adjoining. The sleeping house site, as well as the intervening space, should be raised or filled up several inches higher than the surrounding ground, to prevent surface water from running in, and also to afford drainage. Set the house on this: 14 × 32 feet, [mine is], high side 9 feet, low side 6 feet, shed roof, of common boards; requiring in all—for siding, roofs, and division—about 1,400 feet of common lumber, and a few pieces of scantling or straight hard wood poles to nail to and support the roof; then add six or eight inches of sand or sawdust to the floor and the intervening space, and you will have no mud."

When but few pigs are kept, or it is desired to keep up a small number for some particular purpose, they can in spring, summer, and early fall in many cases, be kept advantageously in small portable pens, which can be moved a few feet every day or two; by doing this the pigs can have the benefit of fresh clean earth and grass continually.

For easy handling, such pens should be light, and are best made of pine lumber, the size of the pens varying according to the length of the boards used, from 10 to 16 feet, and these may be 4, 5 or 6 inches wide—the latter being much the best for strength.

Instead of nailing the lumber to small corner posts, we find it better to make four separate panels, nailing the lumber firmly with wrought nails, to cross-pieces or cleats, of good 6-inch boards, as long as the pen is to be high, three to each panel, and when set up, keeping secured by some sort of flexible fastening.

When nailed together at the corners, the frequent moving of the pen wrenches and breaks the nailed corners loose, and the pen becomes a wreck, a result which cannot occur when the parts are jointed.

If a pen 14 or 16 feet square is built, it is sometimes convenient to have an extra panel, which will fit down in the middle of it, between cleats, which will at once convert the one pen into two of half its size.

These pens should be provided with a convenient

trough, and some sort of temporary roof, over one end or corner, at least sufficient to afford a good shade at all times of the day, which, with plenty of water, is indispensable.

We have found a movable pen or two, quite a necessity in the summer season, but cannot recommend any pen, that is so light and airy as this, for cold weather.

It frequently happens, on a farm where machinery is used, that four wheels may be found, from 6 to 24 inches in diameter, that may be fastened to the corners of the movable pen, on which it may be moved with facility from place to place, without much effort, or, suitable wooden wheels, of any size or number, can be made of the transverse sections of a solid hard-wood log, and attached to the pen, to enable it to be moved with ease.

On nearly every farm, one or more well constructed movable pens, will be found a good investment, as a few pigs can be kept clean and healthy in these, if moved often on solid ground, with less trouble than in any other way; the farmer who tries them will not readily re-adopt the old-time four-rail-square pen, that stood in the same place for a dozen or more years.

In whatever style the pen may be built, we would impress on the builder the convenience and importance of having the troughs level, with cross-slats on top, six or eight inches apart, and arranged so that feed can be poured into their entire length from the outside of the pen. These assist in the more equal distribution of the feed, enable each animal to secure its share, prevent the stronger from monopolizing and fouling the trough, by standing lengthwise in it, and also enable the attendant to feed without being jostled, or charged upon, by the always importunate swine.

Feeding a dozen or more hogs, by pouring slops into one end of a long open trough, is excellent for two or three of the strongest animals, but the others usually have to stand back, and be content with so much, or so little, of the feed as their more powerful companions reluctantly leave, for want of more capacious stomachs.

Troughs are much more durable if made of good sound oak, or other hard wood, than of pine, as hogs sometimes get into a habit of gnawing them for the taste of something that has soaked into the wood, and a pine trough is, in this way, soon destroyed.

CHAPTER XVII.

SLAUGHTERING, CURING, AND PRESERVING.

Every experiment we know of, that has been made to ascertain whether it was more profitable to the producer to sell his hogs alive, or kill, and cure the pork on the farm, and then market it, indicates that, in most years, the farmer may realize more profitable returns by marketing the cured product. In fact, we have seen but few intelligent farmers who did not admit this, but as they generally need the money represented in the year's hog crop, by the time the hogs are ready for market, they prefer to realize on them at once, rather than assume the risk and wait the longer time necessary to successful curing, especially with the poor facilities many of them possess for this branch of the business.

A lot of uniform, well fattened hogs represent *cash,* any day in the year, at any point in the country; hence the temptation to dispose of them as soon as the proper condition is reached, is exceedingly strong. This, no doubt, accounts in a large degree for the fact, that the bulk of the hog crop raised, is sold on foot to drovers and shippers, to be slaughtered at the immense packing establishments near large cities, and only so many are killed on the farm as are needed for home consumption.

In this, we find the probable reason, why no more attention has been paid to finding out and practising methods in killing and curing of pork, somewhat improved over those of former generations.

We are not aware of anything having been written, nor have we seen practised anything, from which we could infer that the farmers of the present time slaughter and dress their swine in a better way than did their forefathers. The old method of knocking down, cutting into the neck to sever the jugular vein, and pierce the heart, scalding in water not quite boiling, into which a quart of ashes has been thrown "to make the hair slip," scraping with knives, hoes, and iron candlesticks, and then lifting by main strength, the naked, slippery hog to the pole or fixture, from which he is to hang for gutting and cooling, is yet in vogue on nearly every farm.

Those who raise the best of hogs, too often have few conveniences for butchering, and those hurriedly and awkwardly made, generally by the hired man, while the water is heating in the morning. A small expenditure of labor and money would secure such facilities as would render butchering-day much less disagreeable.

After the hog is secured for sticking, either by being caught, knocked or shot down, it should be turned square on its back, and no twist allowed in its neck, so that the sticker will be sure to sever its main arteries, without allowing the knife to penetrate, or injure, either shoulder. We do not deem it best, or even desirable, to pierce the heart, but prefer to let the animal die from loss of blood, which it should do in the space of five minutes, or even less, if the knife has been properly used. When properly stuck, the blood should leap from the gash, in a stream as large as the gash itself, while, or before, the sticker removes the knife.

A barrel or cask is, for many reasons, a poor vessel in which to scald a hog, and any farmer who annually butchers a half dozen good-sized porkers, should provide himself with something less circumscribed and inconvenient, to say nothing of the difficulty of keeping a sufficiency of water at anything like the proper temperature in it.

For farm use, the best scalding vessel we have seen, is a heavy box, 6 or 7 feet long, 30 inches wide at the bottom, and 20 or 24 inches deep, with sides somewhat flaring.

This should have a sheet-iron bottom, well supported on the under side, and be set over a stone or brick foundation, in which there is a convenient chamber for making sufficient fire to readily heat the water in the vessel above, and by which it can be kept thoroughly heated for the length of time required by any number of hogs. At its rear end should be a pipe, or chimney, for smoke, and the sides may be banked up with earth. The description and engraving of the food cooker in Chap. XV. will afford some useful suggestions for the construction of a vat for scalding. The top of the vat should be about 2 $^1/_2$ feet above the level of the ground. On a level with the top, on one side, there should be built a strong platform, about 6 feet wide, and 8 feet long, from which to scald the hogs, and upon which they are to be cleaned, after scalding. At the rear end of this, the ground should be graded up even with the platform, or a sloping platform built, to facilitate getting the hogs on to the main platform, after they have been killed. For convenience in lowering the hogs into, and lifting out of the scalding water, two or more ropes, 8 or 10 feet long, should be secured to the side of the platform next the water, and resting on these, the carcass can be lowered or raised with comparative ease, by two or three men. On the bottom of the vat, there should be some wooden strips or a slatted frame, to prevent the hog from lying directly on the iron bottom, as with much fire in the furnace, the skin would soon cook or burn.

The animal is immersed for a few seconds, and then, by means of the rope, raised out of the water, to allow the air to strike it thoroughly, and then immersed again.

When the hair readily leaves the skin, especially on the head, legs and feet, the hog should be removed from the water as soon as possible, and speedily stripped of every hair. When this is done, the hind legs should be freely cut into, below the gambrel joint, to reach both main cords, under which the gambrel should be entered. The gambrel should be of strong wood—hickory or oak is best—and from 24 to 30 inches in length, according to the size of the hogs, and should be slightly notched on the upper side of each end, to prevent the legs from slipping off.

Posts or forks should be so set, that a strong pole resting on them, will be in part over the platform, about six feet from the ground, and on this the hogs can be hung, and slipped along toward either end, out of the way, after they have been thorougly scraped and rinsed down.

Opening the hogs should be done by some one familiar with such work, and no directions here would be of practical value.

After removing the intestines, the mouth should be propped open with something, and all blood carefully rinsed out of the lower part of the body and neck. The next point, and a most important one, is, to let the carcass, well spread on the gambrel, hang until *thoroughly cooled* in all its parts; unless this is observed, the pork cannot be cured or preserved in good condition, however much pains may be taken with it.

CURING AND PRESERVING.

To cure meat of any kind, it is desirable to have it from animals that, before slaughter, were in a considerable degree matured, or had attained their natural growth. After dressing, as before intimated, the first requisite is to thoroughly cool the carcass, and for this it should hang in a low temperature, for thirty-six or more hours, but on no account should it freeze, especially not after being dressed; freezing its outer surface, surrounds the interior of the flesh with a wall, through which the animal heat, still remaining in and around the bones, cannot escape, and the result will be souring and speedy decay at the centre of hams, shoulders, etc., that outwardly appear in good condition.

Having so large a per cent of fat, side-pork does not readily become over salt, and there is really no danger of injury to any but the leaner portions of the carcass by too much salt; yet where salt is dear, economy would dictate that only so much be used as is actually necessary as a preservative.

Salting with and without brine, are both popular methods, and both are so satisfactory, that we deem one as good as the other.

If brine or "pickle" is used, no danger is apprehended from insects during the pickling process; the brine extracts the blood and other juices from the meat, which rise to the surface, (more rapidly in warm weather), and there decomposing, are likely to contaminate the entire contents of the cask, unless given occasional attention.

The preventive of trouble in this direction is, to occasionally subject the brine to boiling; the impurities will rise to the top, and are to be skimmed off; in this way, the brine may be kept pure, and its strength undiminished, for any desired length of time.

In "dry salting," or salting in barrels, boxes, or piles, without the addition of water to form a brine, it is of the utmost importance that no chance be afforded for flies to deposit eggs, or maggots, or to even come in contact with the meat. If flies have had access to the pork, it cannot then be saved, unless at once put into brine, or kept in a temperature so low the eggs cannot hatch, the latter being not often practicable.

The season of the year, in which meats may be cured on the farm with the best success, is from December 15th to February 15th, the interval between these dates affording two indispensable conditions, viz.: cool weather and immunity from insects and pests.

Pork is cut to suit the demands of the different markets in which it is sold, and the various uses for which it is intended, but the aim should, in all cases, be to have it in such form as to pack snugly, and we repeat, *never pack down until thoroughly cooled throughout.*

Where it is intended to use brine, the meat may be packed in layers; salt, at the rate of eight pounds to each hundred pounds of pork, is to be sprinkled evenly over and around each layer, until the cask is full; then clean rain or other pure water, is poured in, until all the interstices are filled and the meat thoroughly covered. None of the meat should, at any time, be allowed to remain above the brine, and in open casks, or tubs, some attention will be necessary to keep weights so arranged as to hold it under.

Many persons prefer to prepare the brine by adding to the salt some sugar, or molasses, and saltpetre, dissolving these in the water, and pouring the pickle over the packed meat. A very good recipe is as follows: For 100 pounds of pork take 4 ounces saltpetre, 3 pints common molasses, or 2 pounds brown sugar, and 7 pounds clean salt; when thoroughly dissolved, pour over the meat, which it will cover, if properly packed. Many boil the pickle before using it, as the impurities from the salt, sugar, etc., will rise, and can be skimmed off; when this is done, the brine should be thoroughly cool, before adding it to the meat.

Hams and shoulders, to keep well afterwards, should be in pickle from one to two months; the length of time depending on their thickness. For curing them without brine, a favorite recipe is: 12 pounds fine salt, 2 quarts molasses, 1/2 pound powdered saltpetre; when these are well mixed, they will have about the consistency and appearance of damp brown sugar, and will be sufficient for 150 pounds of meat. Rub hams and shoulders thoroughly with the mixture, and lay singly on a platform in a cool, dry place. At the end of the first, and of the second week, rub them again as at first, and then expose to continuous smoke for ten days.

A simpler way, in which any portion, or all, of the hog's carcass can be cured, is to put a layer of, say, half an inch of salt on a platform, floor, or the bottom of a large box, or cask, then a layer of meat, on this a liberal sprinkling of salt, and so on, until all is packed and the top well covered with salt.

Such portions as are not to be smoked, should be stored in brine before insects appear, and the smoked meat may, like the hams of commerce, be covered securely with canvas, and whitewashed, or packed well in bran, dry ashes, oats, or shelled corn. For considerable quantities, packing in tight barrels is a good plan, and for family use, a swinging shelf, with sides and ends covered with wire cloth, inside of which the pieces are hung, is convenient, and is also secure against rats and mice, as well as insects.

The room where any kind of cured meat is to be kept, should be dry and cool, and the darker the better.

The preservative principle of smoke is known as *creosote*. Smoke made by burning corn-cobs is highly esteemed, but those engaged in curing meats on a large scale, consider that the purest, sweetest smoke is obtained from dry hickory sap-wood, stripped of its bark. If the smoking process is too much hurried, the creosote will not have time to penetrate the entire substance of the meat, but ten days steady smoking is, in all cases, sufficient, unless the pieces are unusually large and very thick.

LARD.

Lard is almost a pure oil, of quite a permament composition, for which water has no affinity, and moisture and air have but little effect on it. In the rendering of lard from the tissues in which it is contained, fragments of membrane and particles of animal fibre are intermixed, which would, if exposed to the air, yield to decay; but being surrounded by oil and wholly enclosed, they are kept inactive. Yet, after some time, if abundant, they may become changed and give an odor and taste of decay.

Care should be exercised as to the purity of lard that is designed to be kept, as well as to the exclusion of the air from the vessel. Stone-ware jars (not earthen) are the most desirable vessels for storing lard, which should always be kept in a cool, dry atmosphere.

CHAPTER XVIII.

HOG-FEEDING AND PORK-MAKING.

A great deal of theoretical matter has been published on the subject of feeding animals. Chemical analyses of various feeding stuffs, valuable as they are in showing their nutritive constituents, are not always conclusive evidence of their practical value. There are facts connected with digestion and assimilation which can not be arrived at by chemical analysis. We therefore give a chapter which embodies practical experience based upon scientific knowledge. No one familiar with the agriculture of Ohio need be told of the high position which is occupied by the Sullivants; whether as men of science or as practical agriculturists, whose farming operations have been conducted on a scale unequalled, at least on this side of the continent.

The essay which forms this chapter, is by Joseph Sullivant, Esq., whose wide experience and thoroughness as an investigator, joined to his high scholarly attainments, are well known to the people of Ohio, where he has long been prominent as an officer of the State Board of Agriculture.

The essay appeared in the "Ohio Agricultural Report" for 1869. Its value as a contribution to agricultural literature, and the desire to make it more widely known, are sufficient reasons for giving it a place in the present work.

Having had occasion to inquire concerning the conditions necessary to make hog-feeding profitable, I was somewhat surprised and puzzled at all the discordant answers, and therefore undertook to investigate this subject for myself, and propose here to give the results arrived at, and the basis of my conclusions. In this way my labor may at least become valuable by eliciting the truth from others, who may be induced to enlarge, confirm, or disprove my work.

As to my sources of information, suffice it to say, my materials have been collected and elaborated from various chemical works, agricultural books, reports and transactions of societies, newspapers and periodicals devoted to rural affairs, and conversations with intelligent and practical farmers, and from my own experience.

When we come to know the diverse and varying circumstances under which pork has been made, we no longer wonder at the discrepant opinions and results, and clearly perceive they are owing to the different methods pursued, in which, oftentimes, tradition and caprice have governed rather than an intelligent understanding of the end in view, and the best and most economical means of obtaining it.

The farmer who pens his hogs without shelter from the weather and without bedding, or a dry feeding place, and leaves them to wallow and waddle belly deep in the mire, where the ears of corn sink out of sight, and where the hog has literally to root for his living, cannot expect him to fatten quickly and economically.

Nor can the results be fairly compared to those obtained where attention has been paid to warmth and protection from the weather, a dry feeding place and clean food. And these differing circumstances probably make all the difference of a fair remuneration for food and labor in the one case, or little or no profit in the other.

If we could always command circumstances, we might then reasonably hope for a greater uniformity and reliability of results.

The discoveries in animal physiology, as well as in agricultural chemistry, throw much light on our subject, and point us to the proper path to be pursued, and the direction in which we must look for a rational explanation of the most successful practices *already pursued* by intelligent breeders and feeders

The thorough understanding of the data and principles so acquired, and the proper application of them, will eventually lead us to valuable results.

We may undoubtedly anticipate much benefit from a more thorough diffusion and understanding of the important principles involved in animal physiology and agricultural chemistry, bearing as they do directly on some of the most vital questions in agriculture. There is yet, however, a wide gulf separating theory from practice, although *all* successful practice is but the right application of scientific principles, whether we recognize and apply them, or practice in ignorance of them.

There is one subject of paramount importance so intimately connected with the question of the best and most economical methods of rearing and fattening animals on the farm, as to demand the most serious consideration; I allude to the manure produced and its value in arresting the decreasing fertility of our soils, which is made evident by the gradual, but certain, diminution of the product of our crops, and of which the lessened yield of wheat, in regions formerly productive, is a striking example.

The deterioration of our cultivated lands may be easily accounted for in the fact that for sixty years we have constantly taken from the ground, and, during this long period, returned little or nothing to it. If this condition of things is to be changed, we must alter our methods of farming, and by systematic rotation of crops and by manuring, or by both, endeavor to restore, or, at least, keep in present condition our severely cropped lands, for only by returning some portions of the organic and inorganic matter removed by the crops, can we keep our soil in a fertile state, for, no matter how rich originally or at present, it will, sooner or later, become exhausted unless fed in proportion to the yield required from it. Owing, however, to the great original fertility of our soil, it still yields a fair remuneration for the labor bestowed upon it, and we have not yet reached the point where manure becomes indispensable to the growing crop, as in many places in Europe, where the question is, not how much meat, but how much manure is produced on the farm? And where the profit of feeding consists simply in the value of the manure produced by the animal.

Manure is most valuable in proportion to the nitrogen it contains; and as we propose to feed our hogs on a grain containing twelve (12) per cent of nitrogenized material, the manure should be valuable to us when preserved and applied to our lands. Still, fortunately for us, owing to the cheap production of Indian corn, so far as the profits of feeding are concerned, we may leave the manure so produced entirely out of consideration, and I proceed to the main object of the investigation.

WILL IT PAY TO FATTEN HOGS ON CORN ?

In answering this question, the first and most important consideration is that of food; and the *value of equal weights* of the different kinds used for fattening purposes will depend upon the proportion of nutritive material in each, and the cost of production.

Without going into detail as to the ultimate elements, we shall content ourselves with adopting the classification of the proximate principles of food into

NITROGENOUS AND NON-NITROGENOUS.

The first representing the plastic material or flesh formers, and the last the heat and fat givers; classing these last together because the surplus carbon not required for maintaining animal heat and respiration is stored up in the tissues in the form of fat.

It has been proven by direct experiment, that both the nitrogenized and non-nitrogenized elements must exist in due proportion in the food to maintain *any* animal in a healthy and growing condition, and if it were fed exclusively on one or the other it would pine and die.

However, it is highly probable that if the nitrogenous elements existed in many articles of food in less quantities than is actually found to be the case, they would still be sufficient for the wants of the animal organism; for a very considerable portion of the nitrogen ingested in the food passes away in the excreta without assimilation, but at the same time adds additional value to the manure.

The following table gives the proportion of this necessary element in one hundred (100) pounds of the different substances that are or may be used in the fattening process, and also the non-nitrogenized or fat giving principles, and the total amount of carbon:

TABLE NO. 1.

Table of the Chemical Composition of some Principal Articles of Food.

EXPLANATION.—The column of "Heat and Fat Givers" signifies—I. Starch; II. Sugar; III. Fat or Oil.

Name.	*Water*	*Flesh formers.*	*Heat and fat givers.*	*Equivalent of starch.*	*Mineral matters.*	*Total carbon.*
Barley	15.1	8.0	I. 74.0 III. 2.0	78.8	0.9	38.69
Beans	12.0	26.0	I. 57.0 III. 2.0	61.8	3.0	40.84
Buckwheat Seed	......	10.7	I. 52.3 II. 8.3 III. 0.4	58.48	1.4	31.74
Cabbage	89.42	1.45	I. 7.01 III. 0.08	7.2	0.12	3.89
Carrots	86.5	1.3	I. 6.3 II. 5.0 III. 0.15	11.3	0.80	6.11
Clover (Red).	81.01	4.27	I. 8.45 III. 0.69	10.1	1.32	6.785
Clover (White)	79.71	3.8	I. 8.14 III. 0.69	10.27	2.08	6.607
Cotton-seed Cake (Decorticated.)	9.28	41.25	I. 16.45 III. 16.05	54.4	8.05	46.0
Indian Corn	12.0	12.0	I. 68.5 III. 7.0	85.3	1.5	41.72
Linseed Cake	10.05	22.14	I. 39.1 II. 11.93	67.1	7.25	41.7
Mangold-wurzel.	Dry.	3.0	II. 73.0	69.0	6.3	32.2
Milk (New)	87.2	4.0	II. 4.6 III. 3.5	12.5	0.7	6.687
Milk (Skimmed.)	88.6	4.0	II. 4.6 III. 2.0	8.8	0.77	5.532
Oats	12.2	18.0	I. 52.5 III. 6.5	68.6	2.54	46.8
Peas (Dry)	15.0	22.6	I. 58.5 III. 2.0	63.3	2.5	39.35
Parsnips	85.1	1.4	I. 10.0 II. 2.5	12.4	1.0	6.245
Poa Pratensis Timothy.)	67.14	3.41	I. 14.15 III. 0.86	16.21	1.95	8.93
Potatoes	75.0	1.4	I. 22.5 III. 0.1	22.7	1.0	11.468
Rye (grain)	15.0	8.8	I. 62.7 II. 2.5 III. 2.9	71.2	1.36	39.9
Turnips	91.1	1.2	I. 3.2 II. 3.0	6.2	1.5	3.39
Buttermilk	89.1	4.0	II. 4.6 III. 1.5	7.6	0.75	5.147
Lucern	69.95	3.83	I. 13.62 III. 0.82	15.58	3.61	8.98
Bread	48.8	8.2	I. 44.5 III. 1.0	46.9	1.5	26.93

The farmer has here a wide range from which to choose, and, knowing the cost of production or market price per one hundred (100) pounds of each, can determine which to select as the most advantageous for his purpose.

If the plastic material, or flesh-formers, be assumed as the basis of value, then equal weights of the grain and seed foods will stand in the following order: Cotton-seed cake (decorticated,) beans, linseed cake, peas, oats, Indian corn, rye, buckwheat, barley; but on the basis of fat and heat givers, they stand, first: Barley, Indian corn, rye, peas, oats, beans, buckwheat, linseed cake, cotton-seed cake. Taking the whole of nutritive matter, they range in the following order: Indian corn, barley, beans, peas, rye, oats, buckwheat, linseed cake, cotton-seed cake, potatoes. Estimated according to the total amount of nutritive material, there is not much difference in the theoretical value of several of these substances, but Indian corn heads the list, and, containing in itself all essential elements for the growth and fattening of animals, we shall adopt it as our standard of value and comparison.

Measured, then, by the theoretic value, one hundred (100) pounds of corn are equal to the weights, as exhibited in the following table:

TABLE NO. 2.

In feeding value 100 pounds of corn equals—

Barley	103	Peas	106	Red Clover	665
Beans	103	Potatoes	360	White Clover	665
Rye	117	Mangold-wurzel	665	Timothy grass	298
Oats	118	Parsnips	618	Lucern	598
Buckwheat	122	Carrots	721	Cabbage	1018
Cotton cake	117	Buttermilk	508	Skimmed milk	721
Linseed cake	119	Fresh milk	865	Turnips	1236

Although it appears from the first table that cotton cake, beans, peas, and linseed cake, contain more of flesh givers than corn, and might very advantageously be fed to young and growing animals, yet, upon the whole, Indian corn stands pre-eminent as the cheapest material accessible to our farmers, and the question now arises—

HOW MUCH PORK IN A BUSHEL OF CORN?

In determining this we shall first consider the composition of corn from a theoretic and chemical view, and then, taking results obtained from the vital processes occurring in the human subject, apply them by analogy to the hog, which, of all our domestic animals, most nearly resembles man in his digestive apparatus.

Looking only at the chemical composition of corn, and separating it into flesh formers and heat and fat givers, at twelve (12) per cent of the first and forty-one (41) per cent of the latter, there would appear to be nearly thirty (30) in the bushel of corn, to be transformed into an equal quantity of pork, through the organism of the hog. But I shall presently show that, whatever the value of corn by the chemical standard, it *is not* all transformed into pork, and therefore there is not thirty (30) pounds to be obtained from a bushel of corn.

It has been determined by competent observers and experimenters who have carefully investigated the subject, that a certain amount of nitrogenized and non-nitrogenized matter, or flesh formers and heat and fat givers, representing the carbonaceous material, is required to keep an adult man of one hundred and fifty (150) pounds weight in good condition; that is, neither increasing nor diminishing in weight, under moderate labor, vital. physical, or mental. As the hog performs no brain work, and is supposed to be almost in a state of rest while fattening, he will certainly require no more of the above elements than does the man, and most probably less. But assuming for him the same amount, it will be amply sufficient to keep a hog of the weight of 150 pounds in as good condition as the man. But if the hog is to fatten likewise, he must have an additional amount of food, over and above that which is merely sufficient to furnish the material consumed in respiration, animal heat, and the restoration of all waste produced by the vital processes.

Before demonstrating what this amount of extra food must be, I premise that the hog is to be sent to market at 300 lbs. weight.

As he increases from 0 to 300, it is evident his mean weight is 150 lbs.; and if we can determine how much corn is required at this weight, not only to restore the daily waste, but to fatten him one pound per diem in addition, we will have solved the problem of the number of pounds of pork in a bushel of corn.

Dr. Edward Smith, an eminent writer and experimenter, is a high authority on vital statistics, and was employed by the English Government to examine and report upon the foods of the laboring classes.

He states that the actual quantity of carbon contained in the food of English work-people, according to the severity of the exertion, is from 30 to 38 grains per pound of body weight. He also says that 28 grains of carbon to each pound of body weight gives the measure which, when united with the proper amount of flesh formers, is sufficient to keep a man of 150 lbs. in good condition under moderate exertion.

Now, as has already been said, the hog, increasing from 0 to 300 lbs., his mean weight is 150, and the amount of carbon necessary at *this* weight will give the mean or average amount required daily for his whole life of 300 days.

Then 150, the mean weight of the hog, multiplied by 28, the number of grains of carbon daily required, gives 4,200 grains, or 9 ounces of carbon, to supply the waste, and keep him in condition; and 22 ounces, or a little less than one and one-half pounds of corn, will furnish the necessary elements.

But to fatten the hog a pound a day, he will require, in addition, 16 ounces flesh and fat material, which will be furnished by two pounds of corn. Thus, 2 lbs. or 32 ounces, contain 12 per cent of flesh formers, and gives $3^{84}/_{100}$ ounces of this material, and the same 2 lbs. containing 41 per cent of carbon, furnish $13^{12}/_{100}$ ounces, and 3.84x13.12=16.96 ounces, or material for a little more than one pound of pork; and therefore 54 ounces, or 3 lbs. and 6 ounces of corn, is the average daily ration while making three hundred pounds of pork in three hundred days.

As 3 lbs. and 6 ounces are contained in 56 lbs., or one bushel, 16 $^{59}/_{100}$ times, there are consequently 16.59 lbs. of pork in one bushel of corn, according to the data here given.

And if the amount assumed to restore the waste in the hog and keep him in condition be correct, then there cannot be made more than the 16.59 lbs., because the elements would be wanting. The amount assigned for waste is certainly high enough, most probably too high; and if we take the amount of carbon and flesh formers simply to keep a man of 150 lbs. in condition when in a state of rest, and modify our statement, the result would be 2½ ounces of flesh formers and 7 ounces of carbon derived from 14 ounces of corn; but two pounds, or 32 ounces, being still required. for the fattening process, we have, altogether, 46 ounces contained in 896 ounces, the weight of a bushel of corn 19½ times; equal to 19½ lbs. of pork.

I have found from a careful examination of experiments in feeding, but not herein set forth, that usually not more than one-third of the food is returned in the form of flesh, even in well conducted experiments; and 3 into 56 lbs., or one bushel, gives $18^{2}/_{3}$, and the mean of 16.59, 19.50, and 18.63 gives such a close agreement of theory with the best practice, that I conclude it is very nearly correct, and that chemistry and physiology have answered our question satisfactorily, or at least fixed a limit beyond which it is not likely we will be able to pass, unless under exceptional circumstances, and the pork from a bushel of corn will not exceed twenty pounds, and will approach or recede from this according to circumstances.

Shelling, grinding, and cooking, the corn cannot increase the existing amount of elements, and has for effect only to render the matter more soluble and digestible, and make the approach to the figures given more probable, than if the corn was fed in the whole and raw state.

But it has been well observed, "in every case in which life is concerned, it is not at once to be concluded that, so much material being consumed, there will be uniformly and necessarily so much product." There are so many modifying circumstances to vary our results, that it is not probable our practice will ever give constant uniformity or perfect coincidence with theory, or the chemical constituents of the food we employ in stock feeding. And, although we may to a great extent master the circumstances under our own control, there still remain unexplained difficulties, arising from the inherent differences belonging to special breeds and constitutions of the animals we have to deal with, as well as the anomalies we have to encounter whenever we attempt to apply theory and chemical principles to living organisms and vital functions, which perhaps, for a long time to come, will continue to baffle our best endeavors and prevent uniform and constant results.

However this may be, the conclusions drawn from the scientific principles I believe to be entirely trustworthy, and are satisfactory, to myself at least, as determining, not only the possibilities, but the high probabilities, and it now only remains to see how far our chemical view is confirmed or substantiated by the average results in actual practice, obtained from a great number of experiments and records; for it would not be safe to draw general conclusions from one experiment alone, however successful.

We proceed to determine, as well as we can, what answer practice and experiment returns to our question:

HOW MUCH PORK CAN BE OBTAINED FROM A BUSHEL OF CORN?

This is so important a question, bearing so immediately and directly upon the value of corn, that we might suppose it had been settled long ago, beyond all controversy. If such be the fact we find no record of it, and it is here our real difficulty commences; for, as we said in the beginning of this paper, the answers are discordant and apparently contradictory.

I find plenty of opinions and guesses, with loose assertions, but comparatively a very few results based upon actual, reliable, and recorded experiments; and, after a somewhat minute research, I propose now to give the condensed results of my examinations, without going into much detail, remarking, however, that, although finding many records of experiments, I have been obliged to reject most of them, on account of irregularity and want of precision. In most of them the corn has been fed in a mixed state with roots, milk, potatoes, and other substances, as well as, sometimes, whole and raw for part of the time, and then in the form of meal, cooked, and raw; and I retain those only which give precise results on the heads we have selected for examination.

RAW CORN FED IN THE EAR.

Taking the experiment of Clay, of Kentucky, for what it is worth, I remark that I am certain there must have been some error or local circumstance vitiating the result; for 5¾ lbs. of pork from a bushel of corn is much the least I have found recorded in any experiment, and much less than was obtained by Renick and Buckingham, whose hogs roamed at will through a cornfield, wasting corn, and from the very fact of exercise and labor in getting their own food, making far less return than if the same corn had been fed them in a pen.

Buckingham also tried the experiment of feeding corn in the ear to hogs in a pen, and got a return of 8¼ lbs. of pork from a bushel of corn.

Thomas I. Edge, of Chester county, Pa., fed 5 pigs, of the same litter, five bushels of shelled corn, and received 47¾ lbs. of pork, or $9^3/_5$ lbs. from the bushel.

B. P. Kirk fed $49^1/_{16}$ bushels, and had a return of over 12 lbs. of pork per bushel.

An experiment at North Chatham, Columbia county, N. Y., gave a fraction less than 12 lbs of pork from a bushel of corn.

Mr. Ellsworth, of Indiana, had 12 lbs. of pork per bushel from corn fed in the ear.

Marcus E. Merwin, of Litchfield, Conn., fed 95 days, and made 9¾ lbs. of pork from a bushel of corn.

A. S. Proctor, of Illinois, fed 61 days, and gained 10 lbs. of pork per bushel.

Wiseman E. Nichols, Morrow county, Ohio, fed 100 bushels of corn in 63 days, and made from it 1,130 lbs. of pork, or $11^{30}/_{100}$ lbs. per bushel. This corn, however, was simply soaked two days in water.

Mr. Van Loon, of Ill., fed 20 days, and made a fraction over 9 lbs. of pork from a bushel of corn.

Mr. Behmer, of Columbus, Ohio, made 10½ lbs. from one bushel of corn.

Even including Clay's experiment, which, I think, ought to be excluded from any comparison of results, the eleven records here presented give an average of over ten pounds of pork from one bushel of corn, fed in the ear and upon the ground.

An experiment, partly of corn in the ear, which was made at Duncan's Falls, Ohio, in 1859, and communicated to the *Ohio Farmer*, is so instructive in several particulars, that I insert it here in a condensed form.

"Last fall, (1859), I turned my hogs into the cornfield on the 10th of September, after having weighed them all; they were taken out October 23d, weighed and placed in a small lot. During this time, from September 10th to October 23d, they ate down 40 acres of corn, and, estimating it at 40 bushels per acre, the increased weight of the hogs, at 4 cents per pound, just paid 40 cents per bushel for the corn they had eaten. Two days after, or 25th of October, I selected of the lot one hundred hogs, averaging 200 lbs. each; they were placed in large covered pens, with plank floors and troughs, and fed as follows: The corn was ground up, cob and all, in one of the 'Little Giant' mills, steamed and fed five times a day all they could eat, and in exactly one week they were weighed again, the corn they had eaten being weighed also, and calling 70 lbs. a bushel of corn, and pork as before 4 cents gross, it was equal to 80 cents a bushel for corn. The weather was quite warm for the season of the year. The first week in November I tried the same experiment on the same lot of hogs, and the corn only brought 62 cents per bushel, the weather being colder." "Third week, same month, same lot of hogs, and corn fed in the same way, brought 40 cents per bushel, the weather getting still colder." "Fourth week in November, weather still colder, fed as above, and the corn brought 25 cents a bushel. This lot of hogs was now sold and another lot put up, which had been fed in the lot on corn on the cob. This lot was weighed and fed as the last for five weeks in December, and the corn averaged 25 cents; the weather being about the same as in November." "This lot was weighed again in the middle of January, and the corn fed during that week averaged 5 cents per bushel, the thermometer being down to zero. Again the lot was weighed, and they *just held their own;* the temperature being below zero from one to ten degrees." And from the above the writer concludes it will not, as a general thing, pay to feed after November.

An analysis of this experiment shows that the hogs made 10 lbs. of pork to the bushel of corn while hogging it down, September 10th to October 25th.

The first week they were fed on ground corn and cob-meal, steamed, they made the extraordinary amount of 20 lbs. of pork to one bushel of corn. Second week, weather colder, 15½ lbs.; third week, still colder, 10 lbs.; fourth week, weather colder yet, 6½ lbs. of pork to one bushel of corn, and the first lot was sold.

The second lot of hogs was fed five weeks in December, on the same food and in the same way as the first lot, the weather being same as in the last week of November, and the corn averaged but 6½ lbs. of pork to the bushel. In January, the weather being very cold, the corn returned but 1¼ lbs. of pork per bushel; and when the temperature sank to zero and below, the corn returned nothing at all! Certainly a most instructive example, showing how the product ran down from 20 lbs. to the bushel to nothing, from the influence of cold alone, and demonstrating beyond all doubt the advantage and the necessity of warmth and shelter.

Although irregular, I will here also insert a remarkable experiment by S. M. Wherry, Shippensburg, Pa., and communicated to the *Practical Farmer*, December, 1869. Here the object was *growth, not fat;* and this practical experiment is valuable in several particulars. Ten pigs of one litter, Berkshire breed, were fed in pairs, having been equalized as near as possible. They were twelve weeks and four days old at the commencement of the experiment, which continued eight weeks, or fifty-six days.

The first pair gained from five bushels of old shelled corn at the rate of $^{84}/_{100}$ lbs. per day, making 94 lbs. of pork, or $18^{4}/_{5}$ lbs. from one bushel of corn.

The second pair ate 280 pounds, (or 5 bushels), of old corn, ground into meal and cooked, gaining 91 lbs., or $18^{1}/_{5}$ lbs. of pork from one bushel, *but less* than from the whole and raw corn!

The third pair consumed 140 lbs. of meal and 280 lbs. of potatoes, and gained 93 lbs.

The fourth pair, fed on 560 lbs. of cooked potatoes, made a gain of 89 lbs.; showing that cooked potatoes, fed alone, have a little less than half the value of corn.

The fifth pair, fed green corn in the ear, 350 lbs., or 5 bushels, reckoning 70 lbs. to the bushel, and they gained the very extraordinary amount of 100 lbs., or 20 lbs. of pork to the bushel.

During all this experiment, each pig consumed but 2½ lbs of

corn per diem, or the supposed equivalent in potatoes or green corn. This experiment alone, without being supplemented and confirmed by others, is insufficient from which do draw a general application; but, as the writer observes, *is very suggestive*, indicating that pigs not pushed, but steadily and moderately fed, make flesh instead of fat, at the rate of $^{84}/_{100}$ lbs. daily, and that, being so fed, they can do their own grinding and cooking with advantage.

It is evident that the greater the number and the longer the time experiments are continued, the higher is the probability that they approach to a reliable and constant average, and if we admit that the thirteen experiments here set forth, were made on adequate numbers and continued a sufficient length of time, they should have great weight in establishing a general rule, which, in this case, would be that one bushel of corn, (or 56 lbs. of corn), fed on the ear, returns, under ordinary circumstances, ten pounds of pork. But, intending to be cautious and moderate, we shall assume, for comparison and calculation, that one bushel raw and whole corn makes 9 lbs. of pork.

RAW MEAL

is supposed to increase in value over raw corn to the extent of 33 per cent; this is the opinion and statement of the Shakers of Lebanon, New York, after a trial of thirty years. If this increase be true, then, according to our basis of 9 lbs. of pork to one bushel of corn, the corn, when ground, should make 12 lbs. of pork. This agrees with an experiment of Mr. Thomas Edge, making 60 lbs. of pork from five bushels of meal.

And this rate of return coincides with two elaborate and extended experiments—one in England and one in this country.

I give here the result of these experiments by Prof. Miles, of the Michigan Agricultural College, and by Mr. Lawes, of Rothamstead, England; and a full account of these very interesting and instructive experiments by Prof. Miles may be found in the "Ohio Agricultural Report for 1868," and that of Mr. Lawes in the "Journal Royal Agricultural Society of England," vol. xiv.

The experiment of Prof. Miles commenced May 2d, and ended December 15th, embracing a period of 203 days, or 29 weeks, and was made on six grade Essex pigs, two weeks old, and from the same litter, and were divided into two pens of three pigs each. During the first few weeks they were fed on a mixed diet of milk, meal, and a portion of roots, and therefore we select the last period of 20 weeks, during which they were fed exclusively on corn meal. The three best pigs, one from pen A and two from pen B, were killed December 15th, and averaged 145 lbs. each; and, deducting the original weight at the commencement of the experiment, each gained in the total period of 203 days 141 lbs. or $69^{1}/_{100}$ lbs. per diem—during a part of this time, (8 weeks), being fed on a mixed diet. One of the pigs from pen B having died, the other two were fed for 20 weeks on corn meal, and in 140 days gained 205½ lbs., or $98^{69}/_{100}$ lbs., each pig, over their original weight, and at the rate of $73^{1}/_{100}$ per diem for this period. In the 20 weeks 935½ lbs. of meal were consumed, equal to $16^{7}/_{10}$ bushels of corn, and giving a return of $12^{3}/_{10}$ lbs. of pork for each bushel, and requiring 4½ lbs. of meal to make one of pork.

The experiment of Mr. Lawes, of England, commenced February 2d, 1850, with 36 selected pigs in twelve pens, and were fed on several prescribed dietaries. The pigs were 9 to 10 months old, and at the time of selection differed among themselves but a pound or two, and when the experiment began averaged 143½ lbs., but a fraction less than those of Prof. Miles when his were killed, and the two might be considered in the light of a continuous experiment—Lawes beginning were Miles ended.

We select for investigation and comparison pen No. 5, containing three pigs, averaging 143½ lbs., because they were fed exclusively on corn meal.

The experiment lasted 8 weeks, or 56 days, during which time each pig consumed 362 lbs., or $6^{46}/_{56}$ bushels of meal, and $6^{46}/_{100}$ lbs. daily, and gaining $79^{68}/_{100}$ lbs. of weight, or $1^{42}/_{100}$ lbs. per diem, and at the rate of 12 lbs. per bushel; a very remarkable agreement betwixt Edge, Miles, and Lawes.

An analysis of the experiments, both of Miles and Lawes, shows very clearly a *rapid decrease* in the rate of consumption of food to a given weight of animal as it fattens; and, although less food is eaten, it takes more of it to produce one pound of increase, so that, as the animal approaches his maturity of fatness, or, as it is termed in England, "ripeness," he may reach a point where the return in pork will not pay for the corn consumed. This point should be watched for and the pig at once sent to market.

At the conclusion of Miles' experiment, the pigs increased less than two per cent in a week.

Prof. Miles remarks of his experiments:

"In the manufacture of pork the best return of the food consumed will undoubtedly be obtained by liberal feeding during the early stages of growth; and we cannot reasonably avoid the conclusion that the same rule is applicable to *all* animals reared for the purpose of the butcher.

"As animals are employed to convert the vegetable products of the farm into animal products of greater value, the greatest profit in fattening may reasonably be expected from liberal feeding during the period of growth, in which the organs of nutrition are capable of converting the largest amount of material into animal tissues in a given time."

And Mr. Lawes established by his experiment "that the larger the proportion of nitrogenous compounds in the food, the greater the tendency to increase in *frame* and *flesh;* but that the *maturing* or *ripening* of the animal—in fact its fattening—depended *very much more* on the amount, in the food, of certain digestible *non*-nitrogenous constituents."

And this accords perfectly, I believe, with all experience.

STEAMED OR BOILED CORN.

I find a number of experiments in which steamed or boiled corn entered as part of the food, for longer or shorter times, and mixed with other things, and only three experiments conducted wholly on boiled corn; one by Clay, gaining 14 lbs. 7 oz. of pork from a bushel; one by Van Loon, of Illinois, who obtained 18 lbs.; and the other from Montgomery county, Indiana, giving a fraction less than 12 lbs. of pork to the bushel of corn; and all three give an average of a little less than 15 lbs.

The Indiana experiment has most of the elements of time and numbers to make it reliable, and I give some analysis of it.

Eight pigs from one litter were put in a pen when one week old and fed nine months, consuming 220½ bushels of corn, and gaining 2,644 lbs. of pork, averaging a gain of 330½ lbs. each pig, or 1⅙ lbs. each per day for the whole period; and the following tabular statement shows the amount of corn fed during each month, the gain in weight, the number of pounds of pork made to one bushel, and the amount of corn required to make one pound of pork:

No. of Month.	*Amount consumed.*	*Total gain.*	*Pounds of pork per bushel.*	*Pounds corn to one pound pork*
	Bushels.	Pounds.		
1st month..................	15	168	11.20	5.
2d "	24	224	9.33	6.
3d "	26½	272	10.30	5.43
4th "	27	316	11.76	4.78
5th "	29½	352	11.96	4.68
6th "	27	360	13.30	4.21
7th "	26½	350	13.20	4.20
8th "	26	327	12.60	4.40
9th "	21	275	13.00	4.30
		Average..	11.85	4.77

Observe how regular is the increase in weight up to the eighth month of their age, when they averaged 241½ lbs—a regular decrease in the amount of food from the sixth month of feeding, and a diminished quantity of corn to make one pound of pork, instead of an increase, as in Miles' and Lawes' experiments, which goes to corroborate what we have already said, that we meet with some unaccountable anomalies which, as yet, we are unable to reduce to any uniform rule. Perhaps these pigs had not yet reached their full capacity of fatness.

I add here two extracts, one from "Evening Discussions" at the recent New York State Fair, 1867; subject: "Cooking Food for Domestic Animals."

Hon. G. Geddes, of Syracuse, New York, said: "He had thoroughly proved, years ago, that cooking, independent of grinding, at least *doubled the value of food.*"

"George A. Moore, of Erie county, New York, said he had fully satisfied himself that the value of food was *tripled by cooking.*"

I quote from "Transactions of the American Institute, 1864." Prof. Mapes says: "The experiment often tried has proved that 18 or 19 lbs. of cooked corn is equal to 50 lbs. of raw corn for hog feed, and that Mr. Mason, of New Jersey, found that pork fed with raw grain cost 12½ cents per pound, and that from cooked corn 4½ cents."

COOKED MEAL.

I find here, as in other cases, much of assertion, but backed by more of experiment; some claiming, on apparently good grounds, that grinding and cooking the meal thoroughly, doubles the value of the raw corn.

Rejecting here, as elsewhere, the many mixed and irregular experiments, we find that Clay obtained 17½ lbs. of pork from a bushel of corn so prepared; Marsh, of Glen's Falls, New York, 16⅓ lbs.; A. G. Perry, 18 lbs.; Thomas I. Edge, Chester county, Pa., 16³/₅ lbs.; Nathan G. Morgan, New York, 20 lbs.; Buckingham of Illinois, 20 lbs.; Jonathan Talcott, Rome, New York, 17.⁹²/₁₀₀ lbs.; Robert Thatcher, Darby, Pa., made two experiments—one on five very ordinary pigs, getting 16⁸/₁₀ lbs.; the other on five superior Chester pigs, and gained 17⁴⁴/₁₀₀ lbs. from a bushel of cooked meal, and remarks: "The surprising gain for food consumed was the result of very careful feeding, clean and warm bedding, and a tight house."

The average of all these experiments is 17⁸⁴/₁₀₀ lbs. per bushel.

David Anthony, of Union Springs, New York, convinced himself by experiment, that when corn fed in the ear was worth 62 cents, ground into meal it was worth 87 cents, and ground into meal and cooked, one hundred and eighteen (118) cents, the last being 91 per cent better than raw corn.

From an examination of the records at my command, I think that, taking the return of pork from a bushel of corn at nine pounds, there can be no doubt that corn ground into meal and fed, increases in value about 33 per cent over corn fed in the ear. That thoroughly steaming or cooking the whole corn, raises its value to but little less than that of cooked meal, which I estimate at 66 per cent over raw corn fed in the ear.

I arrive at this conclusion, not only from the experiments I have herein set forth, but from an examination of quite a number not here given, on account of their mixed and irregular methods. It is true that grinding, steaming, or cooking the corn can in no wise add a single atom to the elements already existing, and raises its value only by rendering the whole nutritive matter available by making it more soluble and of easier digestion, so that the maximum of nutrition is more readily and certainly obtained.

I conclude that nine pounds of pork from a bushel of raw corn fed in the ear, twelve pounds from raw meal, thirteen and a half pounds from boiled corn, and sixteen and a half pounds from cooked meal, is no more than a moderate average the feeder may expect to realize from a bushel of corn under ordinary circumstances of weather, with dry and clean feeding pens. All this is within the amounts we have shown to be probable and attainable upon our chemical basis.

Higher percentages have been frequently obtained in practice than any we shall now assume as our basis in making practical application of our researches. And if it be true that what has once been done can be done again, there is great encouragement for the feeder to study and master the circumstances that will give the higher results. And in this connection, it is important to consider that animals live constantly in a medium colder than themselves for the greater part of the year, and that the lower temperature continually abstracts and wastes animal heat which, in the fattening process, must be maintained in proportion to the temperature in which they live, and that this heat is obtained from the food which, under other circumstances, would be transformed into fat and stored up in the tissues.

And we can readily perceive that warmth and shelter from the vicissitudes of the weather is not only important, but almost indispensable, and without them we cannot expect the highest return for the food consumed; and of the truth of this the Duncan's Falls experiment is a most striking and instr. ctive example.

Having established the fact from chemical elements, that 16 to 19 lbs. of pork are possible, and that 18 and 20 lbs. are not unfrequent in actual practice, under the circumstances indicated, we shall not be deemed extravagant if we take 15 lbs. per bushel as the basis of our calculations in ascertaining per pound the

COST OF PORK,

which, it is obvious, must depend upon the cost of corn and feeding; and in ascertaining this, we intend assuming such a scale of wages as would in any part of the country secure the necessary labor, supposing, as we do, that it is all to be hired, and that the laborers board themselves; and if our estimates are too high, or if the farmer, with his own labor and teams, can reduce the cost below what we state, it will be easy to correct our tables and make them conform to the reduction, which would only increase the farmer's margin for profit.

We assume the wages of a hired man at $2 per day, and two horses with plow or wagon to be worth the same, or four dollars a day for the whole

TABLE NO. 3.

Showing the cost of raising an acre of corn; one man and team plowing two acres per day:

One acre plowed costs	$2.00
Harrowing 8 acres a day, 1 acre costs	50
Planting with machine 8 acres, 1 acre costs	50
Seed for 1 acre	30
Double shovel plowing, or cultivating 6 acres—1 acre costs 66⅔ cents, or cultivating one acre three times	2.00
Deeper plowing, hoeing, extra labor, or rent, as the farmer chooses, or as the season demands	3.00
Total	$8.30

whether raising 35 or 60 bushels to the acre, the labor being the same—that is, the farmer is obliged to bestow upon his crop during the season a certain amount of labor.

Whatever difference of opinion about the distribution of the items here, the sum total for raising the crop I believe to be ample and ought to command a return of 60 bushels.

TABLE NO. 4.

Cost of Gathering and Feeding.

Husking 33⅓ bushels per day to the hand, at $2.00...... 6 cts. per bu

Wages of man and team, at $4.00 per day, hauling and cribbing 150 bushels.............................. 2.6 cts. per bu.

One man with steam power will shell, grind, steam, and feed 75 bushels per day, wages $2.00; fifteen bushels coal at 15 cents per bushel, $2.25..................... 5.66 cts. per bu.

14.26

Or say.................................. 14 33/100 cts. per bu.

which we will take for our future tables.

TABLE NO. 5.

Shows cost of corn per bushel at $8.30 per acre, and raising 35 to 60 bushels per acre:

35 bushels	23¾ cents.	40 bushels	20¾ cents.
45 "	17¼ "	50 "	16¼ "
55 "	15 "	60 "	13¾ "

By adding the cost of grinding, steaming, and feeding, to that of raising and cribbing, we have the total cost of the corn in

TABLE NO. 6.

35 bushels per acre cost	37.50 cents per bushel.
40 " "	34.83 " "
45 " "	31.66 " "
50 " "	30.00 " "
55 " "	29.00 " "
60 " "	28.00 " "

TABLE NO. 7.

Showing the gross value of a bushel of corn when fed on the cob, or in the form of raw meal, boiled corn and cooked meal, rating the return of pork per bushel at 9, 12, 13½, 15 lbs., and selling from 4 to 10 cents per pound:

Pounds of pork from 1 bushel of corn.	Value of pork from 4 to 10 cents per pound.							
	4	5	6	7	8	9	10	
On the ear......... 9	36	45	54	63	72	81	90	Gross value of a bushel of corn in cents.
Raw meal..........12	48	60	72	84	96	108	120	
Boiled corn.........13½	54	67½	81	94	108	121½	135	
Cooked meal... ...15	60	75	90	105	120	135	150	

TABLE NO. 8.

Showing cost per pound of pork, the number of bushels of corn per acre, cost per busshel of raising and feeding, and return in pork—being given according to our calculations:

Bushels per acre..		35	40	45	50	55	60	
Cost per bushel...		37.50	34.83	31.66	30.00	29.00	28	Cents.
Pounds of pork returned per bushel.	9	4.16	3.87	3.51	3.33	3.22	3.11	Cost of pork in cents, and $^1/_{100}$ of a cent.
	12	3.12	2.90	2.64	2.50	2.42	2.33	
	13½	2.78	2.58	2.34	2.22	2.15	2.07	
	15	2.50	2.37	2.07	2.00	1.93	1.87	

TABLE NO. 9.

Showing the total amount of pork per acre, the number of bushels of corn and return of pork per bushel, being given according to our calculations:

Pounds of pork from one bushel of corn.		Bushels of corn per acre.						
		35	40	45	50	55	60	
On the ear........	9	315	360	405	450	495	540	Total pounds of pork per acre.
Raw meal.........	12	420	480	540	600	660	720	
Boiled corn.....	13½	472	540	607	675	742	810	
Cooked meal.....	15	525	600	675	750	825	900	

If we find the price per pound of pork in Table No. 8 corresponding to any particular yield of corn per acre and pork per bushel, and deduct it from the market price at any given time, and multiply by this difference the number of pounds of pork obtained from the bushel, we have the net profit on a bushel of corn. Thus, at 45 bushels per acre and 13½ lbs. per bushel, we find the cost of pork per pound to be 2.34 cents. Supposing pork to be selling at 6 cents per pound, the difference is 3.66 cents; multiplying 13½ lbs. (the yield per bushel), by which we get 49.4 cents as the profit per bushel of corn. If, as before, we find the price of pork in Table No. 8, and deduct from market price, and multiply by this difference the number of pounds of pork per acre, as found in Table No. 9, corresponding to any given yield of corn per acre, and pork per bushel, we have the net profit per acre from pork. Thus, we find by table No. 9, at 45 bushels per acre and 13½ lbs. per bushel, the amount of pork per acre to be 607 lbs. Multiplying this number of pounds by 3.66 cents the difference between cost and selling price, we have $22.21 as the profit per acre of corn.

We have already satisfactorily shown from chemical data above that, after allowing a sufficiency of the elements to restore the daily waste and keep a hog in good condition, there is enough in the corn to bring him from 0 to 300 lbs., at the rate of 15 lbs. of pork per bushel of corn. And practice has shown that there is more than we have assumed in our calculations, and adhering to our maximum of 15 lbs. as one we believe to be easily attainable, and supposing also that the feeder will strive for the higher result, we have prepared a table to show what profit he may expect for his corn with good cultivation, and getting a return of 15 lbs. of pork from one bushel of corn.

TABLE NO. 10.

Selling price of pork per pound in cents.	Whole cost of corn per bushel according to product per acre, at—						
	35	40	45	50	55	60	Bushels.
	Cents. 37.50	34.83	31.66	30.00	29.00	28.00	Cost per bushel.
4	22.50	25.17	28.34	30.00	31.00	32.00	Net profit per bushel.
5	37.50	40.17	42.34	45.00	46.00	47.00	
6	52.50	55.17	58.34	60.00	61.00	62.00	
7	67.50	70.17	73.34	75.00	76.00	77.00	
8	82.50	85.17	88.34	90.00	91.00	92.00	
9	97.50	100.17	103.34	105.00	106.00	107.00	
10	110.50	115.17	118.34	120.00	121.00	122.00	

It appears from our first and second tables, given in a former part of this paper, that, from the chemical elements, there is but little difference in the fattening value of several of the foods there given, but, in so far as they contain more of the phosphates and flesh formers than corn, they could be very advantageously fed to young and growing animals; but the cost of producing equal weights of these must, after all, determine their economic value in the fattening process.

And now, having satisfactorily to ourselves, at least, set forth and established the close agreement of theory with the best practice, not by guesses and loose opinions, but by solid facts and experiments we might here leave the subject for each one to secure the results we have shown to be attainable by the methods best suited to his own circumstances and according to his own notions. But, in consequence of important questions which now arise, we must pursue the subject a little farther, even if it lead us, for the moment, from all well-established facts into the field of hypothesis and conjecture, for we have not here any recorded experiments to assist us in determining a question of much practical importance—

THE RIGHT AGE AT WHICH TO FATTEN A HOG?

Whether it is better to keep him as a store or stock animal, in moderate order and growing condition, on grass and clover with a little corn during winter, until he is matured in growth, at 12, 18, or 20 months old, and then in three or four months feed him up to 400 or 500 pounds, or to winter him only and fatten him in the spring; or is it best to push the pigs from birth and feed them up to 300 lbs. at nine or ten months old?

In order, if possible, to get some light on this point of our investigation, let us take two pigs from the same litter, as near alike as possible, subject them to the same treatment and the same food, terminating one experiment at nine months and the other at eighteen. Then with pigs littered, say April 1st, let them run with their mother on grass and clover until October 1st, a period of six months, or 183 days. It will be reasonable to assume they will make three-fourths of a pound of daily growth and increase for that period, or weigh 138 lbs. each.

We will now take pig A and put him up to fatten, and, as three months or thirteen weeks are amply sufficient to ripen a hog, we will full feed him that length of time, or 92 days. We also desire to bring him up to 300 lbs.; and, as he already weighs 138 lbs., there remain 162 to be added, and, if our estimate of 15 lbs. of pork from one bushel of corn ground into meal and boiled be correct, he must eat 10 $^4/_5$ bushels of corn and get a daily increase of one and three-fourths ($1\frac{3}{4}$) pounds, and so, having arrived at 300 lbs., we dispose of him.

Pig B, also, at the end of six months, or the first of October, weighs 138 lbs., same as pig A, but, instead of being put to fatten, we wish to continue him to May first, or 212 days, and, gaining at the same rate as before—that is, three-fourths pounds daily—as from April to October. During this period, from October to May, he consumes $11\frac{1}{4}$ bushels of corn, gains 159, and then weighs 297 lbs. Again, he pastures from May to October, gaining, as before, 138 lbs., and now, at October first, when he is put up to fatten, weighs 435 lbs., and, being fed for the same period as was A, or 92 days, and making the same increase, he now weighs 594 lbs., and has eaten altogether a little over 22 bushels of corn and twelve months of pasture. Pig A, for six months pasturage and 10 $^4/_5$ bushels of corn, returns 300 lbs. of pork, while pig B, for twelve months pasturage and 22 bushels of corn, returns but 594 lbs. of pork—being a difference of six (6) pounds of pork and one-fifth of a bushel of corn in favor of feeding two hogs like A rather than one as B, making the same amount of pork and returning the money invested in one-half the time.

From the fact that both Lawes and Miles found, as the hog approached ripeness, or full maturity of fatness, the quantity of corn to make a pound of pork increases, and the time also, it may be that our suppositious cases are very near the truth; I think they are, and that it will take less food to make 600 lbs. of pork from two animals than from one. And the rates of increase and total weights given of the animals is rather strengthened and corroborated by the fact that from an examination of the weights given of several hundred extra heavy hogs (upwards of 350,) of the age of 20 and 22 months, very few reached 600 lbs., and none made an increase of one pound a day for that whole period.

There are many experiments proving that hogs of 18 to 22 months frequently increase during the fattening process at the rate of 2½ to 3 lbs. a day, and even more; and that young hogs are very often made to weigh 300 lbs. and over at the age of 9 to 10 months.

There is no doubt a certain proportion betwixt muscle and fat while feeding, which will be found to give the most advantageous results; but it is so apparent that, to obtain great weight in any animal, we ought to have a good supply of bones and muscle to begin with, and a sufficient frame-work on which to build and lay the fat, that I think it would be advisable to devote the first few months of the pig's life to *growth* rather than for *fat-making*, and to this end S. M. Wherry's experiment, on page 183 furnishes a good example. And it will be well to remember that Miles' pigs, with an insufficient frame-work to carry more, were ripe at seven months old, with a weight of 145 only pounds, having been *pushed* from the start.

Having shown how much pork is to be expected from a bushel of corn, prepared and fed in various ways, we will devote a brief space to considering the expense of preparation. It will be observed that in estimating the lowest cost price of pork, we assumed 15 lbs. as our maximum return from a bushel of corn.

But in obtaining this result we have shelled, ground and cooked our corn meal with steam power, and it may be said, with truth, perhaps, that this can only be applied economically on a large scale—say to feeding upwards of 250 head—to feed less would hardly justify the necessary outlay for machinery and apparatus, and we must try some other plan more suitable for smaller operations.

From an examination I am satisfied it will cost upon an average 15 cents to have corn shelled and ground, including toll and transportation to and from the mill. That is to say, taking our yield of nine pounds of pork from raw corn, and 12 from raw meal, we must get 15 cents from the three additional pounds, or five cents per pound for the pork, to pay the cost of grinding.

It is obvious that this pork must sell at some price greater than this to afford any profit on the three pounds so produced, and to gain even five cents per bushel above the product, and nine pounds per bushel, we must get 6⅔ cents per pound for the pork. But now, having our corn ground into meal, let us proceed to cook it, which I estimate will cost seven cents per bushel on a moderate scale, with simple apparatus; and 15 cents, the cost of grinding, added to seven cents, the cost of cooking, equals 22 cents.

From corn so prepared, we expect a return of 15 lbs. of pork per bushel of corn, and a gain of six pounds over raw corn, producing but nine pounds. These six pounds have cost 22 cents, or 3⅔ cents per pound, and it is evident that, for every cent per pound above this cost that the pork brings, we gain six (6) cents more than when getting but nine pounds per bushel. Then, at 6⅔ cents for pork, our profit would be 18 cents for these six additional pounds per bushel.

Suppose now, instead of incurring the expense of grinding, that we steam or cook the whole grains of corn, at the same cost as the meal—seven cents per bushel—and gain thereby 4½ lbs. over the product of raw corn (to wit: nine pounds,) then, at 6⅔ cents per pound for pork, our profit would be 23 cents per bushel for these 4½ additional pounds, and in like proportion for any higher selling price for pork.

In all calculations of expense throughout this paper, we have intended to make ample and liberal estimates.

It is plain, from a comparison of the above statements, that, although getting but 13½ lbs. of pork from a bushel of boiled or cooked corn, it is yet the most economical method of preparing the corn on a moderate scale, and affords not only a possibility, but a high probability, of a larger return than we have given.

And, fortunately the apparatus required is simple and inexpensive, for any vessel with a capacity to turn into steam 26 gallons of water per hour is sufficient, if we assume that corn has the same capacity for heat as water, to raise 10 bushels of corn to the boiling point in one hour and keep it there, and furnish a daily ration for 60 hogs. But it is evident the corn must be kept some time at the temperature indicated to cook it. No doubt on many farms there already exist the pans and brick arches used in the making of sorghum molasses; and these pans, with some alterations and inexpensive additions, would, no doubt, answer an admirable purpose. So, also, will a large kettle set in an arch, answer to cook corn for 10 to 30 hogs. The corn, whether cooked in the pans or kettle, should be shelled and placed in trays with stout wire bottoms just close enough to hold the grains of corn; and, placing these trays, if need be, one on top of the other, just above the water in the pan or kettle, let *all* be covered and steam away. I think that for about 75 or 80 dollars, an apparatus on this principle can be made, sufficient for 150 hogs. In any apparatus for cooking or steaming the food, one square foot of pan or kettle exposed to the fire, is the *minimum* space capable of evaporating one gallon per hour—1½ feet is better.

It is propable the corn could be ground on the farm with horse-power, cheaper than we have estimated, if the feeder will invest in a mill and necessary power.

Opinions differ as to any real value in feeding the cob ground with the meal; some attaching great value to the method, others rejecting it altogether.

Chemical analysis of the corn-cob gives six to ten per cent of matter that may be rendered, by long maceration and boiling, capable of assimilation by the animal.

I myself believe there is not nutriment enough in the cob to pay for getting it out; but an occasional feed of cob meal would be of service, for in the fattening process, a certain amount of inert matter seems not only to be beneficial, but to be absolutely required by the hog, and it is, no doubt, this instinctive want and necessity, that induces the hog to eat coal, rotten wood, and even clay and dirt.

Having now considered the various methods of preparing and feeding corn, there yet remains one subject to be discussed which is of too great importance to be ignored or overlooked in any scheme of pork-making, I allude to

THE VALUE OF GRASS AND CLOVER.

We have already mentioned it; but, in the absence of any carefully conducted experiments on this point, it is somewhat difficult to determine the pork-making value of grass and clover, as compared with corn. I find great differences of opinion as to the number of hogs an acre of good grass or clover will support during the season; the number varying from three to six—the higher number being assigned to an acre of *good clover*.

Of course the number *must* depend upon the quantity of grass or clover, whether it be thick or thin, and also a good, moderate, or poor crop. In this dilemma let us see if theoretic statements will help us in the solution of this question.

We will assume, to begin with, that one acre, with a good set of timothy and clover, occupying the ground in equal proportions, will give a product of 12,000 lbs. during the season. We think this a moderate estimate, for the reason that it requires less than one ounce of green food per month from each square foot during five months of pasturage. Suppose the average of the hogs, when turned on to grass, to be 125 lbs., and that it be the fact, as has been frequently stated, that an animal requires three per cent daily of his live weight in dry food, or its equivalent in green food, to keep him in a growing and fattening condition, then 7½ lbs. of grass and clover will be consumed by one hog daily from May to October, or 153 days, or 1,146½ lbs. during this whole period. Then it is evident the acre of grass and clover will support as many hogs as 1,146½ is contained in 12,000 lbs. (the product of one acre,) or 10½ hogs, nearly! But we prefer to base our calculations on the data given in a previous part of this paper, that it requires one and one-third pounds of corn to maintain a hog of 150 lbs. in condition merely, and of course requires a corresponding portion of green food to do the same thing; and if, according to our Table No. 2, it takes 6.75 lbs. of clover to equal one of corn, then 1.33 lbs. of corn, (the amount to keep the hog in condition), requires nine pounds of green clover, or an equivalent, to supply the daily waste in the animal organism, and of course an additional amount is necessary to increase the hog in weight; and if we take the increase at one-half pound daily, then 6.75 lbs. more of clover is needed, or 15.75 altogether; but as timothy (of which an equal portion of our green food consists), is in value to clover as 298 to 675, a less amount, or eleven pounds, will suffice than if feeding clover alone. But as some is wasted and trampled down, we think a daily allowance of fifteen pounds to each hog is none too much.

Fifteen pounds of green food, which we have determined as the ration to sustain the hog and fatten him one-half pound daily, is contained in 12,000 lbs., (the product of one acre), 800 times, and would support one hog for 800 days, or 5¹/₅ hogs one hundred and fifty-three days, or five months, from May to October, the period of pasturage. Omitting the fraction, our five hogs increasing one-half pound daily for 153 days, we have a total return in pork of 382½ lbs. from one acre of timothy and clover, and its value can be compared with the amount of pork produced from an acre of corn in Table No. 9.

I estimate the cost of getting a good set of clover and timothy at four dollars ($4) per acre, and that we will have two seasons of pasturage from it; and dividing this cost into two years it will be but two dollars for our 382½ lbs. of pork, or a fraction over half a cent per pound; or, assigning to our grass and clover pork the lowest selling price in our tables, or 4 cents per pound, it gives us $382\frac{1}{2} \times 4 = \$15.30$—and, deducting the cost of the grass and clover, leaves us a net profit of $13.30 for one acre of our pasture. Of course all this is hypothetical, and each one must determine for himself how nearly these calculations are correct. I believe they are within the truth, and will be exceeded in actual practice.

If any one takes the trouble to compare the values of pork and corn on our data of 9, 12, 13½ and 15 lbs. of pork from a bushel of corn, it will be found that, at nine pounds, one pound of pork must bring six and two ninths ($6^2/_9$) times as much as one pound of corn to make the pork equal in value to the corn—at 12 lbs. per bushel one pound of pork must bring 4½ times as much as one pound of corn—at 13½ lbs. per bushel the pound of pork must bring $4^1/_{10}$ times the price of the corn, and at 15 lbs. per bushel the pork requires to be $3^2/_3$ times the value of one pound of corn.

Finally, after a careful and somewhat extensive examination and analysis of quite a number of experiments, regular and irregular, of all the various methods of feeding corn, including a wide range of country and seasons, I find, upon the whole, that, amidst the apparently discrepant and contradictory statements, quite uniform and accordant results have been obtained under similar circumstances. And, notwithstanding the subtle influences of life and the vital processes may continue to evade us, and may never be brought entirely under our control, and made subservient to our purposes, yet, aside from all this, we have the power of perfect command over many of those circumstances, which do undoubtedly exercise a most important influence over the young and growing animal—such as foods in various quantities, forms, and proportions, regular feeding, cleanliness, warmth, and shelter from the weather; and last, but not least, a judicious selection of the breeds and aptitudes best suited to our wants.

And I conclude, upon a review of the whole subject, that it will pay to fatten hogs on corn alone, when properly prepared, and it will be easier and cheaper if a portion of the pork be made on grass and clover.

Where the farmer prepares for pork-making, and pursues it with system and regularity, I believe it will pay him better than to sell his corn, (no matter what be the market price), even at his own door. And especially I think will this be found true by those so situated as to be obliged to haul their corn any distance to market, which increases the cost of the corn 5 to 15 cents, according to the distance to be traveled.

My investigations have led me to some unexpected conclusions, but, having no theory to begin with, I have simply followed where truth seemed to lead, determined to collect and tabulate facts and be guided by them alone, avoiding all mere opinions and assertions.

If we have proved anything, it is, that it is possible and comparatively easy to get 50 per cent more for corn than we now do for all the millions of bushels fed to hogs in the process of pork-making. Sustaining in this industry alone a loss of millions of dollars annually, the question of how much pork in a bushel of corn is *not* an insignificant one.

It strikes me that the different State Agricultural Societies could engage in no more beneficial work than to arrest the enormous losses of our wasteful feeding processes, by the dissemination of correct information, and by a series of well-conducted experiments lend their powerful aid to elucidate so important a subject.

CHAPTER XIX.

THE EFFECTS OF COLD ON FATTENING SWINE.

EXPERIMENTS MADE AT THE KANSAS STATE AGRICULTURAL COLLEGE FARM, BY E. M. SHELTON, PROFESSOR OF AGRICULTURE.

In the West, a very large proportion of all animals kept for their flesh, are fattened during the most inclement season of the year, and they receive protection that is rarely sufficient to break the force of the wintry blasts. In some cases, the corrals, or feed-lots, are located in a belt of timber, a ravine, or a sink in the prairie, but the shelter is rarely sufficient to affect the temperature of the enclosure.

This western plan of feeding has often been condemned on sentimental grounds, but the facts that stock has generally fed well under this plan, and the business of feeding has been profitable to the feeder, have prevented these objections from having very great influence. With the object of establishing some facts bearing on this point, and having a relation to profit and loss, the experiments herein detailed were undertaken.

In the winter of 1880–1, and again in the winter of 1882–3, ten pure-bred Berkshire pigs of good pedigree were selected. The ages of those employed in the experiment of 1880–1 were as follows :

Pen No. 1..	Farrowed	April 12, 1879	Pen No. 4..	Farrowed	July 4, 1879
Pen No. 5..	"	" 12, 1879	Pen No. 6..	"	" 4, 1879
Pen No. 7..	"	" 12, 1879	Pen No. 8..	"	" 4, 1879
Pen No. 2..	"	July 4, 1879	Pen No. 9..	"	" 4, 1879
Pen No. 3..	"	" 4, 1879	Pen No. 10.	"	March 20, 1879

The three dates represent three different litters.

The ten subjected to experiment in the winter of 1882–3 were of three different litters, all farrowed in November,

1881, and so closely related on the side of sire and dam, as to be practically identical in blood. The pigs employed in both experiments, during the summer preceding, and up to the time the experiment began, were kept in a large pasture-field—mostly prairie grass, but containing a small proportion of orchard grass and alfalfa (lucerne)—receiving two ears of corn per pig each day. The pigs were a remarkably uniform lot, and of very excellent quality.

In both experiments, the pens numbering 1 to 5, inclusive, were arranged in the basement of a warm stone barn, and pens 6 to 10, inclusive, in an open yard on the south side of a close board fence, five feet high, but without other protection, except straw "nests," which were furnished both sets as needed. A single pig occupied each pen, an arrangement necessary to the proper apportionment of feed, and distribution of the results of the experiment. It is safe to say, that the shelter afforded to the pigs kept in open yards was greatly superior to that ordinarily given to fattening pigs in the West.

In the first of these experiments, that of 1880–1, in pens 1, 2, 5, 6, 7 and 10, shelled corn was exclusively fed; in pens 3, 4, 8 and 9, a ration of bran, in addition to the corn, was fed, the amount varying but little from two pounds per day. The bran was fed dry, or mixed with water, to suit the tastes of the different pigs. At first this was eaten with apparent relish, but as the pigs increased in ripeness they seemed to care less for the bran, finally refusing it altogether, and about the eighth and ninth weeks, the bran ration was discontinued.

In the experiment of 1882–3, shelled corn alone was fed in all of the pens. In all the pens of each experiment the animals were fed all the corn they would eat, great care being taken that none was left over in the troughs and wasted, and equal care was taken that none should be insufficiently supplied. The pigs were fed twice daily, at 8 A. M. and at 4 P. M., the feed being weighed out accurately to each pig at every feeding. If at the time of feeding the previous feed had not been consumed, the surplus was removed, and a proportionate reduction made in the amount of the next feed. All of the pigs received whatever water they required.

In order to see the effects of variations in temperature, the readings of Fahrenheit's thermometer, in the barn and at the pens in open yards, were recorded every morning at 8 o'clock in both experiments.

All of the pigs were weighed at the close of each week, a little before the time of the first feeding of the week following.

In table No. 1 is shown in pounds and decimals of a pound the weight of each pig at the beginning of the experiment, the total gain, the total gain per cwt., and the average gain per cwt. in the experiment made in 1880–1.

TABLE NO. 1,

SHOWING THE WEIGHT OF EACH PIG AT THE BEGINNING OF THE EXPERIMENT, AND AT THE CLOSE OF EACH WEEK, THE TOTAL GAIN, THE TOTAL GAIN PER CWT. OF EACH PIG, AND OF THE TWO SETS.

Date.	*Week of Experiment.*	*Pigs kept in warm pens in the barn.*					*Pigs kept in open pens in the yard.*				
		Pen 1.	Pen 2.	Pen 3.	Pen 4.	Pen 5.	Pen 6.	Pen 7.	Pen 8.	Pen 9.	Pen 10.
Nov. 1, '80	Begin'ing of Exper't	272	240	258	275	226	244	229	249	252	285
Nov. 8, '80	First.....	281	257	267	294	238	253	239	260	259	292
Nov. 15, '80	Second...	296	266	285	309	251	263	245	269	278	313
Nov. 22, '80	Third....	313	282	297	325	273	287	259	292	293	330
Nov. 29, '80	Fourth...	331	304	319	338	289	304	275	310	308	352
Dec. 6, '80	Fifth. .	349	328	336	357	305	323	288	317	320	362
Dec. 13, '80	Sixth....	365	339	356	376	321	347	306	3[illegible]1	338	387
Dec. 20, '80	Seventh..	389	359	373	396	340	356	321	339	346	392
Dec. 27, '80	Eighth...	400	371	390	409	351	373	336	34[illegible]	355	403
Jan. 3, '81	Ninth...	413	381	399	422	359	382	346	357	356	398
Jan. 10, '81	Tenth....	424	394	410	429	374	384	357	366	356	407
Jan. 17, '81	Eleventh.	435	404	424	439	382	401	366	372	369	409
Total gain.	....	163	164	166	164	156	157	[illegible]37	123	117	124
Total gain per cwt..	....	50.90	68.30	64.30	59.60	69.00	64.30	5[illegible].80	49.30	46.40	43.50
Ave'ge gain per cwt..	....	63.90					52.20				

The remarkable uniformity of this lot is strikingly shown by the "total gain" in both sets, in table No. 1, but particularly in the case of the five pens in the barn, the difference between the greatest and least gain being only ten pounds.

In Table No. 2 the general results of this experiment (1880–1) are given.

TABLE NO. 2.

		Total increase.	Total corn consumed.	Total bran consumed.	Corn consumed for each 100 lbs. live wt.	Bran consumed for each 100 lbs. live wt.	Corn consumed for each 1 lb. of increase.	Bran consumed for each 1 lb. of increase.
Feed, corn.	Pens 1, 2, and 5 in the barn..........	483.00	2,487.50	......	22.03	.....	5.15	.....
	Pens 6, 7, and 10 in open yard	418.00	2,291.00	......	21.64	. .	5.48	.....
Feed, corn, and bran.	Pens 3 and 4 in the barn....	330.00	1,589.00	232.00	21.09	4.13	4.81	0.70
	Pens 8 and 9 in open yard......	240 00	1,386.50	200.00	19.82	4.14	5.77	0 83

A good general view of the results of this experiment may be had by taking as the standard of comparison the cost of 100 lbs. of increase in the two lots of both series, receiving different feed:

100 lbs. of increase, in pens 1, 2, and 5................ cost, 515.02 lbs. of corn
100 lbs. of increase, in pens 6, 7, and 10........... ... cost, 548.08 lbs. of corn.

This gives to the three outside pens, in which corn was exclusively fed, a loss of 33.06 lbs. of corn per cwt. of increase, as compared with pens in which the same feed was used in the barn, and in the 418 lbs. of increase in pens 6, 7, and 10, a loss of 138.27 lbs. of corn, or about six (6) per cent. of the 2,291 lbs. of corn fed in these pens.

100 lbs. of increase, in pens 3 and 4, cost 481.51 lbs of corn and 70.30 lbs. of bran.
100 lbs. of increase, in pens 8 and 9, cost 577.70 lbs. of corn and 83.33 lbs. of bran.

This gives to the two outside pens in which corn and bran were fed, a loss of 96.19 lbs. of corn and 13.03 of bran per cwt. of increase; and in the total of 240 lbs. of increase made in these pens, a loss of 230.85 lbs. of corn and 31.22 lbs. of bran, amounting to about 16 per cent. of all the corn and 15 per cent. of all the bran fed in pens 8 and 9 in the open yard.

It will be observed that the pigs fed outside, besides giving much smaller returns for the feed consumed, in all cases gave less "total gain," and much less "gain per cwt.," as shown in table No. 1, and consumed much less feed than those fed in the barn.

The total loss from feeding in the open yards was quite marked throughout, and the variation in individual cases was considerable. It was noticeable that the quietest animals, the best feeders of those fed outside, endured the severe weather the best, and gave the largest returns for food consumed. These, during the severe weather which prevailed during the sixth, ninth, and tenth weeks, passed much of the time in a condition closely resembling hibernation; they came to their feed during severe weather with great apparent reluctance, and rarely oftener than once each day, during the remainder of the time lying very still, the vital functions manifestly moving at the slowest pace.

The importance of a ration of bran or other coarse feed in connection with corn, for fattening pigs, is frequently urged by writers, on theoretical grounds. It was chiefly to test this question that bran was used with corn in the proportion before detailed, in two of the pens of each of the two series. The value of the bran fed in this experiment may be shown in a brief summary and comparison of the results obtained. In pens 1, 2, 5, 6, 7, and 10, in which corn was exclusively fed, 901½ lbs. of increase cost 4,778.5 lbs. of corn, and in pens 3, 4, 8, and 9, in which corn and bran were fed, 570 lbs. of increase cost 2,975 lbs. of corn and 432 lbs. of bran. That is,

100 lbs. of increase, in pens 1, 2, 5, 6, 7, and 10..cost 530.85 lbs. of corn.
100 lbs. of increase, in pens 3, 4, 8, and 9........cost 521.93 lbs. of corn and 75.78 lbs. of bran.

Or 8.42 lbs. of corn had, in this experiment, a feeding value equal to that of 75.78 lbs. of bran—a fact which seems to show that corn alone can be more profitably used for fattening hogs than a mixed feed consisting of corn and bran.

In table No. 3 is given the weight of each pig at the beginning of the experiment and at the close of each week, the total gain, the total gain per cwt. of each pig, of the two sets in the experiment of 1882–3.

TABLE NO. 3.

Date.	Week of Experiment.	*Pigs kept in warm pens in the barn.*					*Pigs kept in open pens in the yards.*				
		Pen 1.	Pen 2.	Pen 3.	Pen 4.	Pen 5.	Pen 6.	Pen 7.	Pen 8.	Pen 9.	Pen 10.
Nov. 27, '82	Begin'ing of Exper't	252	211	223	214	214	200	227	196	237	204
Dec. 4, '82	First.....	269	222	235	228	228	218	251	216	257	209
Dec. 11, '82	Second...	275	244	257	253	251	234	270	236	271	232
Dec. 18, '82	Third....	293	253	268	262	258	244	278	249	288	246
Dec. 25, '82	Fourth...	309	271	285	275	295	258	289	241	299	242
Jan. 1, '83	Fifth.....	315	279	291	285	277	263	299	259	315	261
Jan. 8, '83	Sixth ...	324	282	305	290	287	262	295	269	321	266
Jan. 15, '83	Seventh.	343	301	319	311	296	278	319	276	338	270
Jan. 22, '83	Eighth...	346	308	330	322	301	283	323	272	344	275
Jan. 29, '83	Ninth ...	356	317	337	334	316	283	334	289	360	286
Feb. 5, '83	Tenth....	373	330	347	346	322	288	337	283	363	282
Total gain.	....	121	119	124	132	108	88	110	87	126	78
Total gain per cwt..	....	48.00	56.40	55.60	61.68	50.40	44 00	48.40	44.40	53.12	38.20
Ave'ge gain per cwt..	....	54.20					45.90				

Table No. 4 shows for each week of the experiment, the average temperature, total feed, the feed for each 100 lbs. of live weight of animal, the total gain, and the number of pounds of feed required for one pound of gain in the two phases of the experiment.

TABLE NO. 4.

		Average Weekly Temperature, Fahr.	*Total Feed, lbs.*	*Feed for 100 lbs. of live wt. of Animal.*	*Total Gain, lbs.*	*Lbs. of Feed for 1 lb. of Gain.*
Pigs kept in warm pens in the barn.	1st Week....	38°	228	19.8	68	3.30
	2d "	33°	293	24.2	98	2.98
	3d "	36°	329	24.8	54	6.10
	4th "	42°	334	24.2	81	4.12
	5th "	32°	312	21.5	32	9.76
	6th "	21°	277	18.8	41	6.80
	7th "	29°	294	18.9	82	3.58
	8th "	19°	272	17.1	37	7.32
	9th "	27°	263	16.1	53	4.94
	10th "	20°	274	16.8	58	4.72
Pigs kept in pens in open yard.	1st Week....	31°	243	21.9	87.0	2.80
	2d "	22°	327	26.9	82.0	3.98
	3d "	21°	341	26.0	62.0	5.50
	4th "	29°	333	25.3	19.0	17.55
	5th "	15°	322	11.8	73.0	4.41
	6th "	5°	274	19.0	16.0	17.50
	7th "	18°	279	19.2	68.0	4.11
	8th "	12°	248	16.6	16.0	15.46
	9th "	15°	249	16.3	55.0	4.61
	10th "	2°	226	14.4	1.0	226.00

From the table No. 4 it will be seen that:

In pens 1, 2, 3. 4, and 5, in the barn, 2,878 lbs. of corn gave 604 lbs. of pork, and
" " 6, 7, 8, 9, and 10, outside 2,844 " " " 479 " " Or,

In the warm pens, 1 lb. of pork cost $4^{76}/_{100}$ lbs. of corn, while
In the outside " 1 " " " $5^{93}/_{100}$ " "

Again—In pens 1, 2, 3, 4, and 5, in the barn, one bushel of corn produced $11^{76}/_{100}$ lbs. of pork.

In numbers 6, 7, 8, 9, and 10, outside, the same quality of corn produced $9^{43}/_{100}$ lbs. of pork.

Or, in other words: of every bushel of corn fed in the five open pens, an amount sufficient to make $2^{33}/_{100}$ lbs. of pork was used up in keeping the animal warm.

The effect of very cold weather upon fattening pigs is still more strikingly shown by comparing the results obtained in the two sets—barn and outside—during the four weeks of lowest temperature, namely, the sixth, eighth, ninth, and tenth weeks of the experiment, as follows:

In the warm barn, 1.086¾ lbs. of corn gave 190 pounds of pork.
In the open pens outside, 997 lbs. of corn gave 88 lbs. of pork.

Or, in the warm barn, during the severest weather, 1 lb. of pork cost 5.71 lbs. of corn.

While outside, during the severest weather, 1 lb. of pork cost 11.32 lbs. of corn.

It is found that during the period of highest temperature, when mild winter weather prevailed (the average temperature in the barn was thirty-seven degrees, outside twenty-six degrees), the pigs in the barn made a much larger increase in weight (thirty-one pounds) than those in open yards, upon less corn (sixty-one pounds), giving a pound of increase for about four-fifths of the corn required by the pigs in the exposed pens. In the period of *greatest* cold this variation is much more marked, as shown above, except in the total corn consumed, the pigs in the barn consuming eighty-nine and a half pounds more of corn than those kept outside. The small amount of feed consumed outside, during this period, is safely attributable to the severe weather that prevailed during the time referred to.

The principal results of this experiment may be shown in a few brief comprehensive statements :—

(1.) In the warm barn, 2,877½ pounds of corn gave 604 pounds increase in the weight of the pigs, while in the open yards 2,844 pounds of corn gave 479 pounds of increase.

Or, in the exposed pens, the cost of one pound of increase was almost twenty-five per cent greater than the cost of one pound of increase in the warm barn.

(2.) Besides giving less of "total gain" and "gain per cwt." in every pen, during every week of the experiment, the pigs fed outside gave much smaller returns for feed consumed, but this was especially marked during the weeks of lowest temperature.

Thus, during the three weeks of greatest cold, the pigs in open yards required 17.50, 15.46, and 226 pounds of corn for each pound of increase, while in the warm barn, during the same three weeks, 6.80, 7.32, and 4.72

pounds of corn respectively were expended for one pound of increase.

(3.) In this, as in the experiment made two years ago, I have observed that the quietest pigs, the "best feeders," suffered least from cold, ate the best, and gave the largest returns for feed consumed.

(4.) The fluctuations in the weekly gain were very much greater in the pens in the open yards; but, as shown in Table No. IV., whenever little gain or a positive loss was sustained—as in the pens 8 and 10, during the fourth week, and pens 6 and 7, during the sixth week—an enormous gain was made during the week following, even though the temperature continued low, as though the animals were making a determined effort to recover lost ground.

(5.) The fluctuations in the total feed consumed, or in the amount of feed consumed for each 100 pounds of live weight of animal, were not great in the different pens, or in different weeks of each pen, although these fluctuations were greatest in the "outside" pens, the smallest amount of feed being consumed during the coldest weather. It is worthy of remark, however, that in the weeks following, those showing the least gain in flesh or the greatest loss, when the largest increase was made, as stated above, the increase in the amount of feed was inconsiderable: in some cases nothing. Thus in pens 6 and 7, in the sixth week, and in pen 8 in fourth and eighth weeks, the pigs lost 1, 4, 8 and 4 pounds respectively, while in same order consuming $55\frac{1}{2}$, 48, 61 and $43\frac{1}{2}$ pounds of corn. During the week following, when the same pigs gained in weight, 16, 24, 18, and 17 pounds, the enormous gain was made at a cost of $55\frac{1}{2}$, 52, 60 and $46\frac{1}{2}$ pounds, respectively, of corn.

Surely these facts can lead to but one conclusion, that it will pay to give pigs warm quarters during the feeding period. May we not reasonably infer from these same facts, that *all* classes of domesticated animals, for whatever purposes they are kept, will give the largest profits when well housed and made comfortable?

CHAPTER XX.

FEEDING FOR FAT AND LEAN.

It can scarcely be denied that during the period of say thirty years in which general attention has been paid to improving and largely rearing improved breeds of swine, the tendency has constantly been towards producing animals that yielded a maximum quantity of fat or lard with only a minimum of lean meat or muscle. This is easily traceable to the fact that the principal food of the swine in the regions where they are most raised is Indian corn, which is a fat-former unequaled by any other grain grown or used on American farms. Among other results of feeding almost exclusively generation after generation of animals a food so ill balanced or imperfectly adapted for a general maintenance ration, are an impaired vitality, a weakened bony structure, decreased fecundity, and in the matured carcass a ratio of fat to lean meat much greater than the average consumer finds profitable to buy or palatable to eat. Among the subjects that the better class of hog-raisers are now coming to consider as of importance are the treatment and foods, or combinations of foods, best adapted to economically produce pork with such an increased percentage of lean, or judicious admixture of lean with fat, as shall be most healthful, most palatable, and most eagerly sought by those upon whom their market depends, and best for their families. Helping to the solution of such problems has already become recognized as a part of the legitimate work at the different State Experiment Stations and Agricultural Colleges, and a valuable beginning in that particular line has been made by Prof. J. W. Sanborn, at the Missouri Agricultural College, and by Prof. W. A. Henry, director of the Agricultural Experiment Station at the University of Wisconsin. The experiments of each produced a great similarity in results and are very interesting. In making a condensed report of his effort in that direction for this volume, for which he will have the thanks of the reader as well as the author, Prof. Henry says:

"Once knowing that foods of different compositions do affect the frame and flesh of animals differently, and how and why, we are in position to go ahead and build up a better system of swine husbandry than we now have. Knowing corn to be a universal hog food and often used almost exclusively by many of our farmers, and further knowing that chemistry shows that corn is excessively rich in the carbohydrates or heat and fat-formers, while it is low or poor in protein and ash elements which go to make up bone and muscle, we thought to feed it exclusively to one lot of hogs that we might see the effects it produces. To another lot it was thought best to feed a ration excessively rich in protein, which makes it the opposite of the first ration. To this end we made up a ration of shorts sweet skim milk and a little dried blood. Dried blood is not often used as a food, but is wonderfully rich as may be supposed in the same elements as dried beef. Dried blood, skim milk and shorts are each comparatively rich in protein, so it will be seen our feed for the second lot was rich in muscle-making food, and if there is anything in what chemists tell us about foods, our pigs, having such widely different rations, should show it in their bodies, if the character of the food makes any difference.

"Out of a litter of eight pigs, six were selected, even in size and form, for the trial, when they were 100 days old. Up to the beginning the pigs were all fed alike, from the same trough, a mixture consisting of shorts, corn meal, skim milk and buttermilk. The pigs were cross-bred Jersey Reds and Poland-Chinas. At the beginning of the trial the six were divided into two lots of three each, and to Lot A was fed a ration consisting of one part of dried blood, six parts of shorts, and fourteen parts of sweet skim milk by weight. To Lot B was fed all the fine ground corn meal they could properly consume. Water was freely provided for each lot, and each had the run of a small yard back of the feeding pen in which exercise could be taken; all went on with remarkable uniformity from first to last, with no accident of any kind during the whole period of 136 days. The following shows in a condensed form the amount of food consumed by the two lots during the trial of 136 days:

LOT A, FED FOR LEAN.

Amount of sweet skim milk consumed	3,302 lbs.
Amount of shorts consumed	1,415 1/7 lbs.
Amount of dried blood consumed	235 6/7 lbs.

LOT B, FED FOR FAT.

Amount of corn meal consumed	1,690 lbs.

"The digestible matter in the food fed to the two lots was as follows:

	Protein.	*Carbohydrates.*
Total digestible matter fed to Lot A	428 lbs	833 lbs.
Total digestible matter fed to Lot B	153 lbs	1,193 lbs.

"It will be seen that each lot received about the same number of pounds of actual food, but that the proportion of the protein to the carbohydrates varied greatly. Protein goes to make muscle, though it may be used for heat and fat in the body. The carbohydrates (starch, sugar, etc.) cannot make muscle in the body of an animal, though they may save it from waste and decay, but are used for maintaining the bodily heat and for making fat. Our corn-fed hogs then were fed a very fattening food, while the other lot were given a large amount of muscle- (or lean meat) making material. Here we have our feeds so widely different in character that the effect should be very evident in the carcasses of

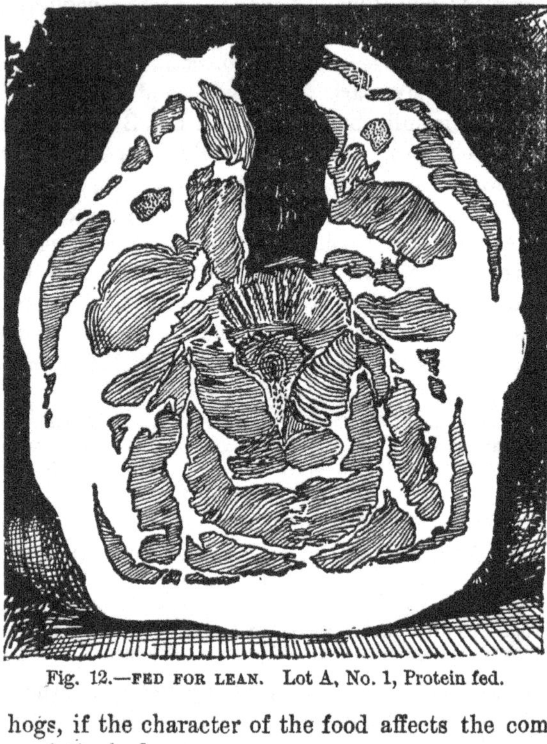

Fig. 12.—FED FOR LEAN. Lot A, No. 1, Protein fed.

the hogs, if the character of the food affects the composition of the body.

"The hogs were slaughtered Nov. 8, 1886, a skilled butcher assisting, every operation being conducted with great care and precision. After taking the live weight of each animal, it was killed by slow bleeding, and the blood caught and weighed. The viscera were taken out and each organ weighed and the dressed hogs hung up to cool and stiffen.

"Upon being taken to the block each dressed hog was laid on his back, and first the head was severed, next the body was cut square across between the fifth and sixth

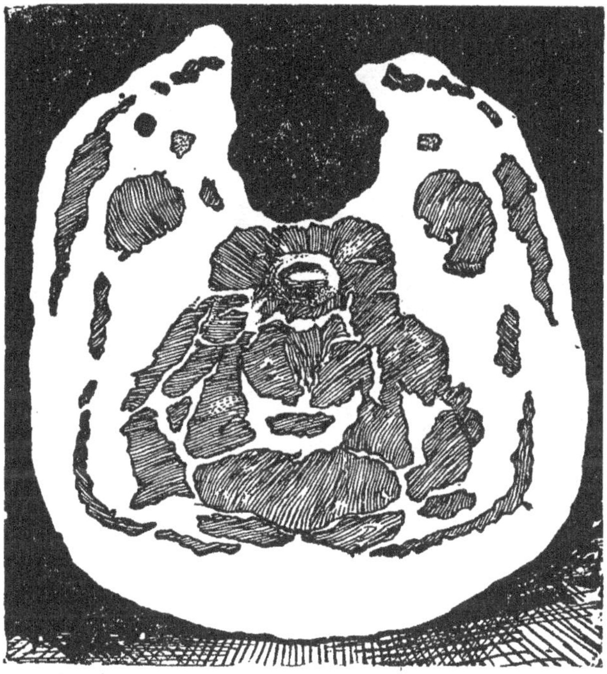

Fig. 13.—FED FOR FAT. Lot B, No. 1, Carbohydrate fed.
Figs. 12 and 13 show in cross section the proportional size of the muscles (lean meat) in the necks of hogs of each lot.

ribs, and again at the loin or small of the back. A painter was employed to sketch the appearance and disposition of the fat and lean meat as exposed by the cuts. Fearing the painter was not exact enough, a photographer was employed for the same purpose, and we were thus enabled to preserve for future reference and study that which would have otherwise soon been lost.

"The illustrations which are herewith presented show the proportion and disposition of the fat and lean in some of the cuts. We present six, three of each lot.

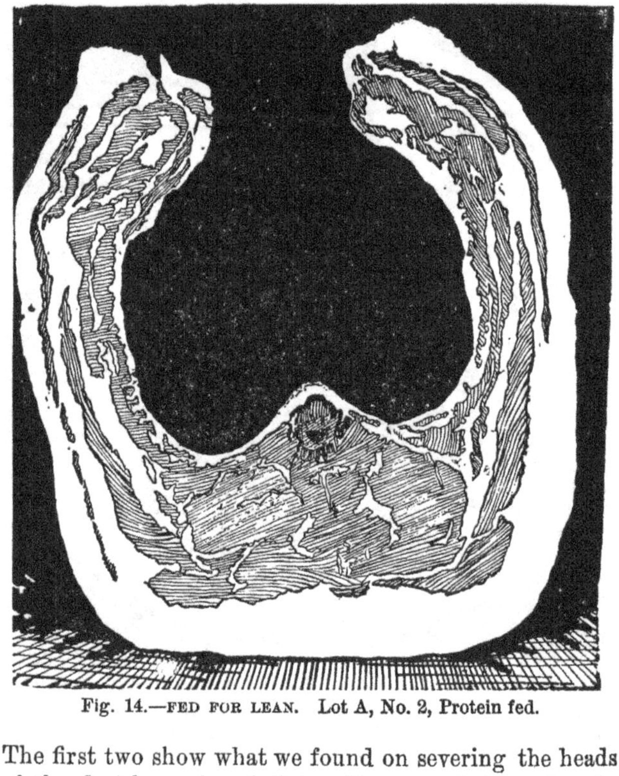

Fig. 14.—FED FOR LEAN. Lot A, No. 2, Protein fed.

The first two show what we found on severing the heads of the first hog of each lot. The second two show in the same way the cuts made between the fifth and sixth ribs of the hogs numbered "two" in each lot; while the last two engravings show the loin cut of the hogs numbered "three" of each lot. In each of the engravings the dark shaded parts represent lean meat or muscle, while the fat is shown by the white parts. As in cutting across the body at the three places named we cut square across most of the muscles, the reader can see the relative size of each muscle in cross section in two hogs of

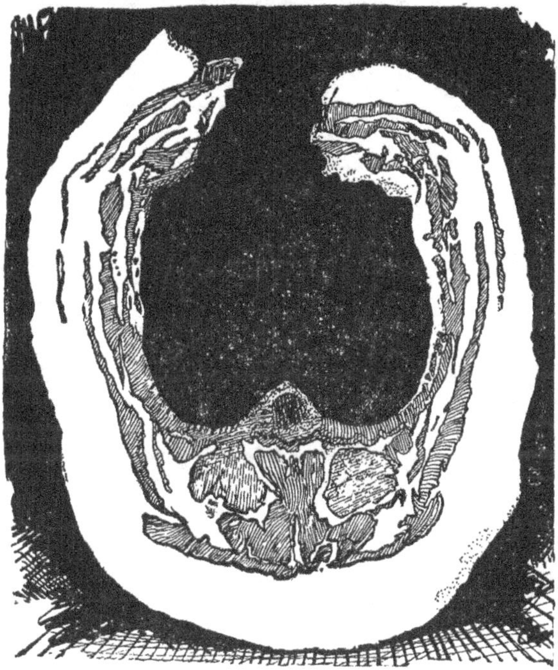

Fig. 15.—FED FOR FAT. Lot B, No. 2, Carbohydrate fed.
Figs. 14 and 15 show in cross section the proportional size of the muscles (lean meat) over the heart of hogs of each lot.

each lot. The illustrations are made from the dressed hogs lying on their backs.

"The reader is asked to give these illustrations more than a passing glance—to study each. It will be seen in each case the muscles (red or lean meat) of the protein fed hogs are larger than the same muscles of those fed the ration rich in carbohydrates. Even the muscles of

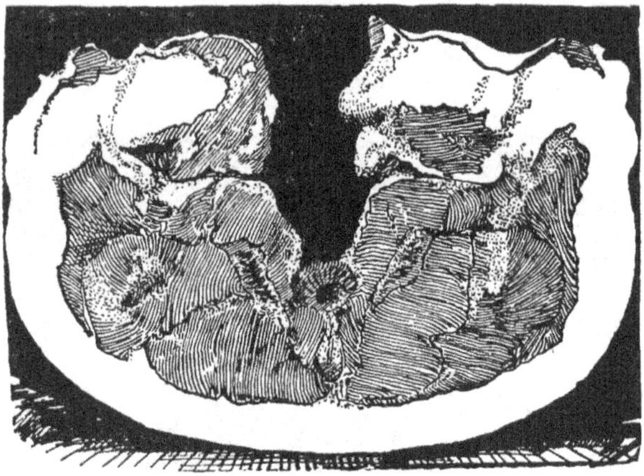

Fig. 16.—FED FOR LEAN. Lot A, No. 3, Protein fed.

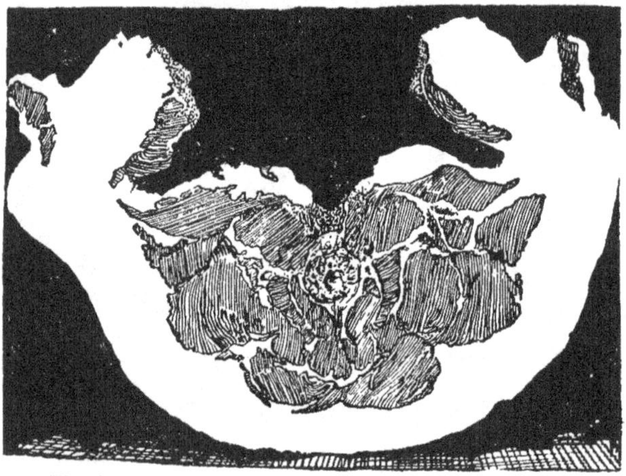

Fig. 17.—FED FOR FAT. Lot B, No. 3, Carbohydrate fed.
Figs. 16 and 17 show in cross section the proportional size of the muscles (lean meat) of the hogs of each lot cut through the small of the back.

the neck are stronger, as shown in the first two cuts. On the back over the heart, the muscles of Lot A show far less fat between them than of Lot B. The most remarkable difference, though, is in the small of the back, where it will be noted that Lot A has about twice as much muscle as Lot B.

"The viscera of each lot was carefully dissected out and weighed and some most remarkable differences between the two lots were found. The hair was saved and weighed. Each hog was carefully skinned and the skins weighed. The large muscle of the back, also the tenderloin muscles, were dissected and weighed. The bones were freed from tendons and flesh by boiling and the thigh bones were broken on a testing machine, to determine the strength of each. Each bone was laid on two iron edges about a quarter of an inch thick, set four inches apart; a similar iron edge was brought down from above just midway between the two edges below. This plate was crowded down by a lever until the bone broke. In this way we broke five thigh bones of Lot A, and the same of Lot B. We found that the aggregate pressure required to break five thigh bones with the protein fed hogs was 4,550 pounds, or an average of over 909 pounds per each bone; against 2,855 pounds, or 571 pounds per each bone, with the corn fed hogs. Here was a weakening of the bones of over 300 pounds each in 136 days.

"IMPORTANT CONTRASTS IN WEIGHTS.

"The following table gives the most important facts in the case, the weights being of three hogs in each lot.

	LOT A. *Fed for lean.* lbs.	LOT B. *Fed for Fat.* lbs.
Total live weight	669¼	561½
Total dressed weight	541¾	451
Total external fat	150	156
Total lean meat	244	178½
Total weight of kidneys	27	19
Total weight of spleens	16	12
Total weight of livers	146½	109½
Total weight of blood	296	186
Breaking strain 5 thigh bones	4550	2855

"But figures placed in this way are largely lost to the general reader, so I will take the liberty of placing them in a different form :

1. The live weight of Lot A (fed for lean) is 19 per cent greater than Lot B, fed for fat.

2. The dressed weight of Lot A is 21 per cent greater than Lot B.

These differences should be borne in mind in considering what follows.

3. The kidneys of Lot A weighed 42 per cent more than those of Lot B.

4. The spleens of Lot A weighed 33 per cent more than those of Lot B.

5. The livers of Lot A weighed 32 per cent more than those of Lot B.

6. The blood (caught on killing) of Lot A weighed 59 per cent more than that of Lot B.

7. The hair on Lot A weighed 36 per cent more than that of Lot B.

8. The skin of Lot A weighed 36 per cent more than that of Lot B.

9. The large muscles of the back (*Ilio spinalis*) of Lot A weighed 64 per cent more than those of Lot B.

10. The two tenderloin muscles (*Psoas magnus*) of Lot A weighed 38 per cent more than those of Lot B.

11. Thirty-eight per cent of all the meat that could be cut from the carcasses of Lot A was fat, while the fat of Lot B was 46 per cent of all that could be separated.

12. The bones of Lot A were 23 per cent heavier than those of Lot B.

13. The thigh bones of Lot A were 65 per cent stronger with the testing machine than those of Lot B.

"In testing the strength of the bones another remarkable exhibition of the difference in the lots was obtained. By the table it will be seen that the number of pounds pressure required to break the thigh bones of the hog was as follows :

	Pounds Strain Required to Break.		
	First Bone.	*Second Bone.*	
Lot A.			
Number 1	1030	1090	
Number 2	840	790	
Number 3	800	----*	
Total for lot	-------	-------	4550
Lot B.			
Number 1	645	580	
Number 2	600	580	
Number 3	450	----*	
Total for lot	-------	-------	2855

* A ham from a hog of each lot was cut across to examine the meat, and in this way one thigh bone was spoiled for this test.

"We observe an excess in weight of most of the important organs of the interior cavity in the hogs fed for lean over those fed for fat. These differences cannot be accidental, as they are the average of the lots in each case, and the work was too carefully done to have errors sufficient to cover such differences. It will be noted that the liver, kidneys and spleen are all considerably larger with Lot A than with Lot B. A most striking difference is seen in the blood obtained upon killing the hogs. From the three hogs fed for lean we got 18 pounds, 8 ounces of blood, while from the three fed for fat only 11 pounds, 10 ounces. While the blood thus obtained is not by any means all that is in the body of the hog, it is remarkable that we should get so much more from one lot than from the other.

"Before making any deductions we wish to make plain, if possible, that which seems a most important consideration, and one that must be clearly understood before we can use these experiments as we should. All through this discussion, we have carried the impression that we could put lean meat or fat on the hog at will; but can we? Is it not true that in every animal there is a certain limitation to muscular development beyond which it cannot go? The blacksmith or the baseball player develops a large amount of muscle, but the limit is not very high, after all, with them, and probably a man weighing 175 pounds cannot add, either by what he eats or the exercise he takes, over a very few pounds of real meat or muscle to his body; indeed when men "go into training" they reduce their weight as a rule instead of increasing it, getting rid of fat and water in the body. On the other hand, when men have a tendency to laying on fat, the limit they may reach may double their normal weight. We may say, then, that the possible muscular development of an animal has a narrow limit comparatively, while the possible fatty development has a much wider range.

"We should hold, it would seem, that our hogs which show the best muscular development are only normally developed, or at least have not departed far from the normal, and that whatever we find in them is a condition to be held as a standard, while our hogs which have grown fat and show a variation from the lean hogs are abnormal.

"Having assumed the above as correct we can make a much clearer statement of the deductions which may be drawn from the experiments. The experiments show that when we feed to our hogs a ration rich in carbohydrates but lacking in protein, like corn meal, we will find :

"1. That there is an excessive development of fat not only on the outside of the muscles and beneath the skin but also among the muscles. 2. That the muscles of the body fail to develop to their normal size, especially some of the most important ones, as those along the back. 3. That an abnormally small amount of hair and a thin skin results. 4. That while the brain, heart and lungs do not seem to change in weight, the spleen, liver and kidneys are unusually small. 5. The amount of blood in the body is greatly reduced from the normal. 6. The strength of the bones may be reduced one-half.

"We may conclude that a system of feeding which robs the hog of half its blood and half the natural strength of its bones, and produces other violent changes, is a most unnatural one, and must, if persisted in, end in giving us a race of animals unsatisfactory to all concerned. From parents thus weakened must come descendants that will fall easy victims to disease and disaster. Knowing the facts as here set forth, can we any longer wonder that our hogs are weak in constitution and easily break down when attacked by disease? Nor is this all; the meat from such animals can hardly be of flavor and composition satisfactory to the consumer.

"If even a part of what has been set forth is correct, is it not high time we turned our energies toward better methods? To do this calls for higher thought and better care, but I fully believe no extra outlay of money; rather, I believe, we can feed hogs more profitably by rational methods than by the unscientific and shiftless ways now only too common. First of all, we must see to it that breeding sows are fed a proper ration in which protein compounds form a liberal share. The young pigs must likewise have a goodly allowance of protein, while the mature hogs, when fattening, can be fed a large proportion of carbohydrates, especially if we wish to make a large proportion of lard. The food articles at our command which are rich in protein are skim milk, buttermilk, shorts, bran, peas, green clover, and the like. No farmer can afford to manage his farm with a minimum of these muscle-making foods; they should be supplied abundantly and at a reasonable cost if we will only study to do so.

"Shall we raise less corn, then? Not at all. The corn crop is the best of all we raise, and let the word be "more," rather than less. We need it all, but we must not forget that protein is somewhat lacking in the corn. We may compare our corn to the bricks which go into a building, and the protein food to the mortar which cements the bricks together. He who would lay up bricks without mortar builds foolishly, and his house will tumble. Should he find out his mistake, such a man should not from that date neglect the bricks and turn his whole attention to the mortar. Plenty of good strong mortar and an abundance of bricks are what he needs. We do not want less corn, but we want more clover, more shorts, more bran, more peas, more skim milk, and more clover to bring the highest results.

Without attempting to give any exact rules for guidance, the following statements may not be out of place: During gestation, breeding sows should have only a small allowance of corn, the feed being mainly that which will go to give her young good sound bodies. Such feed would be shorts (middlings or ship-stuff), bran, skim milk, buttermilk and clover. When suckling her young, of course milk is one of the best articles at our command. When weaned, the pigs may get say two parts of milk by weight, one part of shorts and one part of corn meal. A run on good clover would go far to make a good frame. When nearing maturity the ration can be changed more and more to the carbonaceous, and for the last two months, when fattening, the feed can be largely corn, if one desires fat pork, but if lean juicy meat is desired the muscle-making foods must be continued."

In writing of some further experiments he made with other lots of hogs, to see if the results confirmed those previously made, Prof. Henry says that "in general they did." To one of these lots corn meal was fed; to another skimmed milk and corn meal, and shorts and corn meal to a third. His conclusions from what he has seen are that "skimmed milk and corn make the largest hog with the strongest bones; that corn alone makes the next largest hog with the weakest bones; that two-thirds shorts and one-third corn meal make the smallest hog with the most muscle, most blood, and bones very much stronger than the corn alone."

In the experiment by Prof. Sanborn there was fed to one lot of pigs a ration of four parts of ship-stuff (shorts or middlings) to one part of dried blood, this forming a ration excessively rich in protein; to the other lot was fed a ration of corn meal which, as before stated, is excessively rich in carbohydrates. Two hogs of each lot were killed and examined upon reaching maturity, with the results shown in the following table:

	LOT I—*Fed for Lean.*				LOT II—*Fed for Fat.*			
	No. 1.		No. 2.		No. 1.		No. 2.	
	lbs.	oz.	lbs.	oz.	lbs.	oz.	lbs.	oz.
Live weight of pig	138	6½	170	4½	139	15	170	14¾
Heart		7½		8½		7		10
Lungs	1	9½	1	15½	1	15½	1	13½
Liver	3	3	4	½	2	5½	2	9
Spleen		2¾		3½		2½		3
Kidneys		8½		8½		4½		5½
Leaf	2	2	4	10	5	4½	7	13½
Paunch	6	4	5	14	5	4	7	8
Intestines	12	10	11	12½	10	8	11	
Fat of intestines	2	10	3	12½	4	5	4	
Brains		4½		4½		3½		4¾
Fat of body	38	14	50	3	46	4	70	1½
Lean and bone	64		79		58	4	57	11
Hair		11		13		9½		11
Blood and loss in cooling	4	15½	6	11	4	1½	6	

CHAPTER XXI.

THE GRADUAL DISAPPEARANCE OF WHITE SWINE FROM AMERICAN FARMS.

Most of those who were familiar with hog-raising in the United States twenty years ago, are aware that white swine were much the most numerous, and that in many localities those of any other color were so rare as to be regarded almost as curiosities. Since that time, or perhaps more particularly since about 1865–6, the black or black-spotted swine have grown rapidly in popular favor; so much so, in many sections, as to practically displace all others.

Our attention was incidentally called to this fact many times during the year 1881, and in November of that year mention of it was made in a prominent publication devoted to live stock, only to be vigorously combated as a mischievous and exaggerated statement. The vigor of these contradictions caused us to make some effort to ascertain whether the position, as to the disappearance of the white hogs, was or was not really well taken, our own personal observation having been made more especially in Kansas. As to the swine displayed at the two (virtually) State fairs there in 1881, we found that at the exhibition at Lawrence there were about 300 specimens, but one of which was white; that one was a Chester boar shoat, brought by some Illinois breeders, with their display of twenty-four black hogs, in hopes of finding some one in the State who would buy him. At the State fair held at Topeka, the Secretary informed us that there were entered in the Berkshire rings, 368; Poland-China, 350; Essex, 23; Jersey Red, 18; Chester White, 1; total number of entries, 760.

From the Secretary of the Illinois Board of Agriculture and his reports, we learned that at their State fair in 1877, there were 843 entries of swine, and all but 184 of them were entries of Poland-Chinas, Berkshires, or Essex; in 1878, he reported 684 entries, all Poland-Chinas, Berkshires or Essex, but 223; in 1879, he reported 516 entries, 74 of them Chesters, 66 Suffolks, and 376 Poland-Chinas, Berkshires, or Essex; in 1880, he reported 437 entries, of which 269 were Poland-Chinas, Berkshires, or Essex. Secretary Fisher wrote, that in 1881 the entries were, Poland-Chinas, 117; Berkshires, 141; Essex, 57; total black, 315, against 112 entries of Chesters and Small Yorkshires. The Reports of the Indiana Board of Agriculture stated that at the State fair of 1879 there were 297 entries of swine, of which 25 were large white breeds, 28 "Essex and Suffolk," and 4 "Red," against 240 Poland-Chinas and Berkshires; in 1880, there were 314 hogs entered, and 287 were of other than white breeds. Under date of December 8th, ult., the Secretary of the Ohio Board of Agriculture wrote: "Of the hogs exhibited at our fairs for two or three years past, about 70 per cent. were of the dark breeds; the white breeds seem to be rapidly on the decrease."

Prof. L. N. Bonham, of Ohio, a gentleman who knows much of the swine interests of his section, wrote us December 7th:

"In Southern Ohio, I think, white hogs are not so numerous as ten years ago. Occasionally, some farmer, with more enterprise than good management, concludes his swine are not so good, do not make as wonderful growth as some breeders claim in their advertisements of white or red hogs, and accordingly invests in a Chester White or Jersey Red boar. We have had a few such cases in this county, but they do no better than our Butler County Poland-China swine, and the buyers do not continue in the use of them. These new purchases only add to the number of mongrels, of off-color. They are not better feeders nor are they cholera proof, as one breeder claims for his red hogs. So rare are white hogs here, that they are a curiosity."

Of the more recent State fairs in Iowa, Secretary John R. Shaffer wrote:

"The number of entries of dark breeds of hogs at our State Fair of 1880, was 226; of white breeds, 104. Fair of 1881, there were of the dark breeds, 253; white breeds, 110. This would indicate about one-half; but our white hogs, I do not think, would exceed 20 per cent. Poland-Chinas and Berkshires are the predominant breeds, with the Polands in the lead."

As to the great fairs of the North-west, held at Minneapolis, Minn., we wrote to the Secretary, Mr. Charles N. Clarke, who replied:

"The ratio of white to dark hogs exhibited at our fairs the past three years, has been about 2½ to 7½, or about 25 per cent. white to 75 per cent. dark. I judge from observation and experience, that while the white hogs are not to disappear altogether in or from the Western States for many years, they will be bred only in comparatively small numbers. I think while the old, large-boned white hogs are running out, small-boned breeds will work in."

Mr. R. C. Judson, Secretary of the Minnesota State

Agricultural Society, in answer to inquiries, said, December 9th:

"I send you the entries of swine as they appear on my books. Of Berkshires, there were 6 exhibitors; of Poland-Chinas, 8; of Essex, 2; of Suffolks, 1; and of Chester Whites, 2—or, all told, 18 exhibitors of dark hogs, and 3 of whites. As to the number of animals, there were 27 Berkshires, 2 Suffolks, 26 Poland-Chinas, 3 Chester Whites, and 5 Essex, or a total of 58 dark, and 5 white hogs."

Kansas City, Mo., has been for years famed for its Annual Exposition and Agricultural Fair, where breeders of the most approved kinds of live stock have been at great pains to exhibit representatives from their herds and flocks. For several years, Mr. Wm. Epperson has been the Superintendent of the Swine Department of the Exposition, and he makes the statement that the percentage of dark-colored hogs shown there has been about as follows: In 1876, 90 per cent.; in 1877, 85 per cent.; in 1878, 90 per cent.; in 1879, 85 per cent.; in 1880, all were black; in 1881, all were black.

Statements from the St. Louis and other leading fairs showed, relatively, about the same conditions as to numbers as the foregoing, but the stock markets, and not the fairs, are the places where it is practicable to form really correct estimates of the color, quality, and numbers of the hogs that are raised from year to year. The fact that a good many white hogs appear at the fairs may indicate that their owners are either men of superior energy and enterprise, or, to dispose of the stock, they have realized the need of such advertising as fair-going affords them. Kansas City is no mean hog market, and there were handled at its stock yards, in 1881, about 1,000,000 head. At our request, the Superintendent of the Stock Yards, Mr. H. P. Child, made some observations for us, and, Dec. 7th, wrote:

"Fortunately, for my plan, we had quite a heavy run this

morning; and, taking advantage of it, I went through our pens, and counted all the hogs that were from two-thirds to all white, and at the same time tallied the car-loads. In this manner, I found 491 white hogs scattered through 110 car-loads. Our run for the month just passed was 1,678 cars, and 113,132 hogs, an average of over 67 per car. Assuming these to be in the same ratio, gives us 7,330 for the 110 cars. This gives the proportion at 6.66 white, and 93 34 black hogs in every 100 head—a larger proportion than I estimated, my guess being about two to the car, while this shows nearly four. This I consider a very correct estimate and criterion to gauge by, as the hogs that I looked over were received from all points and roads that feed our market. I had not time, or really opportunity, to make separate estimates on localities, but I could see that they varied considerably, in that some few cars were very largely white, as high as 40 head in one car, and from 20 to 30 in several others, while on the other hand I would pass load after load without a white hog in them. This is, of course, for the current year. I have no means of arriving at an estimate on preceding years, other than personal recollection, which would place the percentage in 1871 and 1872 at about half of each, decreasing to about 20 per cent. white in 1874, and a gradual decrease to the present proportion from that time to 1881."

Most of our readers do not need to be told of the amount of business done at the Chicago Union Stock Yards, or of the millions and millions of hogs that pass through them. We asked John B. Sherman, the long-time superintendent of those yards, to give his estimate of the ratio of white to black or dark hogs that had been handled at the yards in 1879, 1880, and 1881, and his statement is this:

"For the years mentioned, I will say, about 90 per cent. of hogs received at the Union Stock Yards were dark colored."

With a disposition to ascertain if the same great ratio of dark hogs would be shown by a later and more extended counting at the Kansas City yards, Superintendent Child, on the 8th of February of this year (1883), instructed his employés at the several scales to keep an accurate and separate account of all hogs weighed, in which the white or red color predominated, and report to him each evening. These numbers, deducted from the total, gave the number of black or dark hogs; the weighing included all the hogs received up to the night of March 7th—one month—and aggregated 108,086 head, of which 5,364 were white, and 737 red, the percentage being 94.36 black, 4.96 white, and .68 red.

In speaking of the matter, Mr. Child said: "My report in 1881 made no account of red hogs, and all that were here at the time were classed with the blacks, so that to show just how much farther the black breeds have crowded out the white now than then, we must add the red to the black again, which gives us 95.04 against 4.96 per cent., or a gain for the black hogs in the year and a half of about one and seven-tenths per cent. I am not able to report, except in a general way, as to the difference in districts or on the several lines of railroad centering here, though the Northern part of Kansas and Southern Nebraska will run somewhat lighter in white than the above, and have very few red hogs, and my judgment is that over half of the latter come from Western Missouri."

That Mr. Child's estimates are substantially correct, we have many times been satisfied by viewing in the yards of the great packing houses at Kansas City, where, in the large droves, amounting to thousands of head, purchased by them almost daily, it is oftentimes difficult to find as many as half a dozen on which the black does not predominate. At the same time, the red or sandy-colored swine, so rare in the West a few years ago, are becoming slightly more common and more favorably considered.

[Personal observation convinces us that practically the same state of affairs exists at this writing—1888. THE AUTHOR.]

CHAPTER XXII.

SOME GENERAL OBSERVATIONS.

ROOTING AND ITS PREVENTION.

Nothing seems more natural to the porcine family than to spend a part of their time in rooting in the ground, and in this way they sometimes do great injury to pastures and meadows where they are kept or allowed to roam. Some way of preventing this has been found a necessity and has been the means of introducing numerous patented articles in the way of "Hog Rings," "Ringers," "Hog Tongs," "Hog Tamers," etc.

The patented rings are usually sold at prices not unreasonably high, but buyers of rings are impressed with the idea that, to use them successfully, tongs, ringers, etc., must be bought also, and for these outrageous prices are charged, which, altogether, makes the ring investment like the little parties that are sometimes made. where it costs one five or ten cents to get in, and as many dollars to get out.

A heavy mattress needle, in a stout handle, or the small blade of a good sharp pocket knife, answers every purpose for making the holes in the animal's nose, and new horseshoe nails, or common No. 12 wire, make rings as good as those covered by patents. If nails are used, they should be hammered into a circular form, preparatory to inserting, and when in, they can be closed with a pair of pincers.

If wire is used, it should be cut into pieces of proper length, put in, and the ends twisted with the pincers, on the awl near the handle. The ends should be well twisted together, and project half or three-quarters of an inch, as the ring will stay in better, and be more of an obstacle in the way of the hog in rooting.

Mr. A. C. Moore describes three ways of preventing swine from rooting:

"1*st*. Place salt and wood ashes in some considerable quantity, at certain places on the ground, so that the earth will become saturated with the salt and lye. It will be found that the hogs will frequent these spots and work out some holes, but thereby satisfy their rooting desires, and the sod will be left undisturbed.

"2*d*. Cut the rim of the snout with your pocket knife, slanting, as to the end and top of the nose, and leave both ends attached, so that the rim will slip up and down when the hog attempts to root. This method, in my experience, is less liable to allow the rim growing fast again, than when the cutting is done by a "hog tamer," provided it is done correctly.

"3*d*. Put two rings in the snout. Buy common iron rings, such as are used by tinners, one inch in diameter, and when the rings are opened sufficiently, and the animal is secured with the usual cord loop on his nose, take a clip punch and make a hole on each side of the center and in the rim of the snout, insert the rings, and force the ends straight."

EAR MUTILATION AND EAR MARKING.

We wish to enter our protest against the practice so common with many farmers, of cutting and disfiguring the ears of their hogs in a brutal manner, under the plea that without it they could not distinguish their own hogs.

It is desirable to have some mark by which the owner may know his own, and a small hole or slit, in some certain place in one ear, need not disfigure it, and yet be just as reliable for identification as the horrible carving and mutilation of both ears.

Well bred hogs have, naturally, fine ears, which add much to their appearance of uniformity and quality, and it seems to a lover of good stock almost like sacrilege to have them mangled, as is sometimes done by savage dogs and more savage men.

SOWS EATING THEIR PIGS.

No one but the breeder who has had the misfortune to see a fine litter of pigs destroyed by their dam—herself perhaps the best sow he has—can have a sense of the annoyance and bitter disappointment such an occurrence involves.

Of such cases a monthly Report of the Department of Agriculture says:

"It is well known that sows not unfrequently attack and destroy their young; or, if prevented from this, will not let down their milk, so that the young pigs necessarily die from want of nourishment. When this condition of things is not caused by a diseased condition of the uterus, it is said that the sow can be brought to terms by pouring a mixture of ten to twenty grains of spirits of camphor, with one to three of tincture of opium, into the ear. The sow will immediately lie down on the side to which the application was made, and remain quiet in this position for several hours, without interfering with her pigs; and on recovery from the stupor, will have lost her irritability in regard to them. The experiment has been tried in Germany hundreds of times, according to one of the agricultural journals, without any injurious effects. It is also said that the eating of pigs by the parent sow can be readily prevented by rubbing them all over with brandy, and making the same application about the nose of the sow herself."

John Boynton, of Stephenson Co., Illinois, describes the way in which he saved a litter of pigs from a vicious sow, as follows:

"I have a fine Chester White sow that has devoured several pigs of other sows, and as she was heavy with pig herself, I expected that when she littered, she would eat them as fast as she could get to them, I watched her closely; she walked up to the first pig and very deliberately opened her mouth wide to take it in. I screamed at her, and she then turned upon me. I continued to menace her until she had to lay down to have another pig; I then got quietly into the pen, and as she was naturally very gentle, I succeeded in getting the pig to her teats, and so I stayed with her constantly, all the while petting the sow, and as fast as the pigs came, would divest them of their entanglements and place them at the teats, which they took right hold of, and before the sow was aware of it, a maternal affection was enkindled in her heart for her offspring. She had, and saved, eight of the finest pigs I ever saw. They are now over two weeks old, and the mother feels all the affection necessary for them. It is well to treat sows gently at all times; then at "littering" time you can do what you please with them."

QUARRELSOME AND FIGHTING HOGS.

When a considerable number of hogs are penned together for fattening, the owner is sometimes much annoyed by finding them disposed to chase and bite one another, and occasionally, to such an extent, that those least able to defend themselves, are chased and worried to death.

We have not been troubled in this way with our own hogs, but as suggestive to those who are, we present the following from "Berkshire," (a most intelligent breeder, withal), of Ridge Farm, Ills.:

"Fifteen years ago, I began feeding a large number of hogs on floored pens, around a flouring mill, and they commenced biting each other. One hog would give another a bite, when he would run and squeal, and each hog he passed near would give him a bite, and thus they kept the poor animal going, until he died. I would go to the pen and stop them, but they would soon commence again.

"I concluded they were feverish, which caused them to be restless, and that they bit each other for the want of something to cool their fever.

"I tried a variety of remedies, and at length fed them some stone coal, which effected a complete cure. I have continued, ever since, to feed my hogs all the coal they would eat, and have never had any more trouble with their biting each other."

THE CONDITION OF SOWS FOR BREEDING.

In our efforts, in years past, to get all the information possible about swine, and their management, we were always confronted with the statement that, a sow tolerably fat at the time of taking the boar, would have but few pigs, and they of such inferior quality as to be worthless, while it was more than likely that the sow and pigs both would be lost.

Hearing this so much, we concluded that what everybody said, must be near the truth.

We are not so positive about this as we were.

Two neighbors raise some model Berkshires, and running a flouring mill, have an abundance of the best of feed, which they use liberally with their breeding sows, keeping them in pretty good bacon order all the time. We used to feel that we were doing a good stroke of missionary work, when we cautioned them about keeping their sows in so much flesh, and that barrenness and failure were sure to follow. They accepted the advice kindly, but continued to feed their sows liberally, and in spite of it all, raised a plenty of good pigs.

Two sows that they thought very highly of, were kept uncommonly fat, and we selected these two as the ones to illustrate our argument, and show by their non-breeding that they had been entirely too well kept.

When the sows farrowed, one had fourteen, and the other fifteen strong pigs, and since then we have labored but very little to convince these gentlemen that "a fat sow won't breed." It has been their turn to laugh.

We cannot doubt that hogs kept and fed at flouring mills, get much nearer a perfect food, than those kept on corn exclusively, and especially is this true of brood-sows and pigs.

IS IT PROFITABLE TO CURE PORK?

Mr. Thomas Wood furnishes us an account of an interesting experiment made by him, as follows:

"A few years ago I made an experiment or two, in order to find out whether it was most profitable to sell my pork or to make bacon of it, and then sell at the prevailing prices.

"I killed a Chester White hog that weighed, dressed, 440 lbs. pork, worth 7c. per lb.—$30.80. When cut up for salting, the different parts weighed as follows:

Hams	116 lbs.
Shoulders	140 "
Sides	81 "
Jowl	16½ "
	353½ lbs.

"Leaving 86 1/2 lbs. weight of lard, chine, or back bone, ribs, face, feet, and other trimmings, worth 5c. per lb.—$4.32.

"The meat, when cured, was hung in a smoke-house for six weeks, then sold and weighed, as follows:

Hams,	106 lbs.,	at.........14c............	$14.84
Shoulders,	130 "	at.........11c............	14.30
Sides,	75 "	at.........10c............	7.50
Jowl,	15 "	at.........6c............	90
	326 lbs.	average 11½c.	$37.54

Value of bacon sold....................................	$37.54
Value of trimmings....................................	4.32
Total....................................	$41.86
Value of the pork at market price..........................	30.80
Profit on making the pork into bacon.....................	$11.06

"This hog was about fifteen months old, and the shrinkage in weight in making bacon was 27 lbs.

"At the same time I killed a pig five or six months old, in order to ascertain the difference in shrinkage.

The pig weighed dressed..	140 lbs.
When cut up, the hams, shoulders, sides, and jowl weighed.....	111 "
Leaving the weight of lard, chine, face, feet, and trimmings.....	29 lbs.

"The meat weighed just the same when taken out as when put in the salt tub; when dried and smoked the same length of time as the other hog, the weight was as follows:

Hams,	31 lbs.,	sold at......14c.	per lb..........	$4.34
Shoulders,	28 "	" ......11c.	"	3.08
Sides,	30 "	" ......10c.	"	3.00
Jowl,	6 "	" ...... 6c.	"	36
	95 lbs.	average 11½c.	"	$10.78
Trimmings, 29 lbs., at 5c. per lb..................				1.45
				$12.23
The pork, 140 lbs., at 7c. per lb., was worth......				9.80
Profit on making pork into bacon................				$2.43

"From this it appears that the shrinkage is proportionately much greater in the pig pork, than in the pork of the older and more mature hog, also that there is a greater proportional weight of trimming."

REPORTS OF REMARKABLE GROWTH.

In the January (1876) Number of the *National Live Stock Journal*, a correspondent published an item stating that Mr. A. Messer, of Mankato, Minn., had just butchered a thorough-bred Berkshire pig, five months and twenty-three days old, that weighed, when *dressed*, 323 lbs.

This was such a marvelous story that we were incredulous enough to doubt it, and took early occasion to call through the same journal, for some further proof than the *ex parte* statement of one (possibly very much interested) individual. Other breeders also insisted that, if such a feat had been accomplished, the parties cognizant of it should certify to, and make public what they knew.

This elicited an affidavit from the man who bred the pig, as to its age, one from Mr. Messer, who raised and fed it, as to its identity, and another from the butcher who dressed it, as to its weighing the 323 lbs. net, all three of which substantiated, in effect, the original statement. After this, the breeders of fine Berkshires throughout the country, who had never raised a pig to half that weight at the same age, demanded to know how such rapid and enormous growth had been produced, and in course of some months it was published to the world in the following language:

"He was kept in a lot 15 × 20 feet, with a few boards laid over one corner, to form a shelter, and under this shelter was a good bed of straw. The pig was kept in these quarters until the weather became cool, when a comfortable little sty was built in one corner, 6 × 6 feet. The pig was fed on the swill from the house, with corn meal stirred in; but had no cooked food whatever, except pieces of bread from the table, which were thrown into the swill.

"He was fed regularly three times a day, and had *all he would eat.* He would eat all he could, then go grunting to his bed of straw—lie down, and continue to grunt. In fact, the most of the pig's time was spent in grunting, eating, and growing."

Although accompanied by proof, this statement surpasses our belief, as it seems beyond the range of human possibilities that such *extra*ordinary pigs can be produced by any such ordinary means, and we take the responsibility of advising our farmer friends, when looking around for extra good pigs to breed from, to discount such stories as the foregoing *at least* 50 *per cent.*

PRIZE ANIMALS FOR BREEDING.

It is a very common practice with farmers and breeders to attend the County, State, and Inter-state Fairs, for the purpose of selecting, from those on exhibition, swine for breeders, and it is considered quite an achievement to attend one or more of the prominent expositions and take home to the farm the pig, or pair of pigs, decorated with the blue ribbon. They look fine, and are fine, but not fine enough to offset the disappointment and chagrin of the credulous buyer, who, after patient effort, fails in nine cases out of ten, to ever produce from them any stock that looks as those did at the fair.

The show-yard may be the best place to see and buy stock for *show* purposes, but not for breeding.

Only the initiated know the various and peculiar methods employed, in fitting up those animals to which were awarded premiums, over such strong competition as they encounter at leading fairs. We recently conversed with a breeder, whose greatest triumph in life had consisted in having premiums awarded to two of his pigs, at one of the great St. Louis fairs.

He said he "scooped" all competitors, and gave the following as some of the methods used to produce such meritorious(?) animals:

"They were fed on beefsteak, cut into small bits, and dropped into new warm milk, as much, and as often as they would eat. They had daily a bath of warm, soft water and castile soap, after which their hair was dressed with olive, or sweet oil."

Premium pigs, produced by such treatment, afterwards getting only common fare, do but poorly indeed, and to expect them to reproduce a family of show pigs, is to cherish a dream that will fail of realization.

Breeders of fine swine, as of fine cattle, frequently sacrifice their best animals for show purposes, and their preparation for this, in a majority of cases, unfits them for thereafter successfully reproducing their kind.

FEEDING COOKED WHEAT.

The following statement, of remarkably rapid gain in weight from feeding hogs on cooked wheat, is given by a correspondent of the *Cincinnati Gazette:*

"On the 4th of August, 1870, I put up 15 hogs, weighing 2,400 lbs., and fed them 5¼ bushels cooked wheat the first week. On the 11th their weight was 2,600 lbs.; gain, 200 lbs., or a gain of 13⅓ lbs. to the hog, being nearly 2 lbs. a day. The next week I fed them 6 bushels of the cooked wheat, producing an increase of 215 lbs., or 14⅓ lbs. to the hog, being a gain of over 2 lbs. per head a day. The third week I fed them 10 bushels of cooked wheat, resulting in a gain of 260 lbs., or 17⅓ lbs. a head, or $2^{10}|_{21}$ a day. The fourth week I fed them 11¼ bushels of cooked wheat, the gain being 320 lbs, or 21⅓ lbs. a head, or a fraction over 3 lbs. a day each. The hogs were then sold and taken away. They gained in four weeks 995 lbs. on 32½ bushels of wheat. In this manner of feeding I received a good price for the wheat, as the hogs were sold at $8.25 per 100 lbs."

HOGGING OFF CORN FIELDS.

The Hon. J. M. Millikin, in the *National Live Stock Journal,* writes as follows:

"I am aware that the people who reside in the East, where grain is high, will be greatly shocked to think that any one would presume to say anything in behalf of such a 'lazy, wasteful, and untidy' mode of using a crop of corn. Indeed, western men can be found who will denounce the unfarmer-like proceeding in unmeasured terms. But let us see if something cannot be said in support of what some may regard as a very objectionable practice.

"In managing our farming operations, there are two things that should not be lost sight of:

"*First.*—We should aim to so manage our affairs as to realize a good profit on our labors and investment; and

"*Secondly.*—To so cultivate our land as to maintain, if not to increase, its productiveness.

"If you have a field of corn of a size suited to the number of hogs you intend to fatten, supplied with water, there is no plan you can adopt of feeding said corn to your hogs that will produce better results than by turning your hogs into the field, where they can eat at their pleasure. As a rule, the weather is generally good in September and October. If so, there will be no loss of grain, while the saccharine juice of the stalks will contribute somewhat to the improvement of the hogs. The expense saved in gathering the corn, and in giving constant attention in feeding, is quite an important item to any man who has other pressing work to perform. Besides, hogs turned into a field for fifty or sixty days are likely to do better than they will do under other ordinary circumstances.

"There is no plan of using the products of a corn field better calculated to maintain its fertility than the hogging-off process. Everything produced off the ground is returned to it; and if the proper mode is adopted of plowing everything under in the fall, the soil will be improved rather than impoverished. This is my theory upon the subject, which is sustained by my experience and observation, and which I have occasionally urged on the attention of others.

"A very few days since I was in conversation with some farmers upon this subject, when a very reliable, careful, and excellent farmer gave this account of his own experience, which I give, with the remark that his statements are entitled to the fullest confidence. He said: 'I have cultivated one field *eleven successive years* in corn, and every fall turned in my fattening hogs, and fed it off. My crops of corn rather increased than diminished. In the spring, after feeding off the corn for eleven years, I sowed the field in spring barley. I had a crop of forty bushels per acre. I plowed the barley stubble under, and sowed the same field in wheat. The next harvest I had a crop of wheat of *forty-two and a half* bushels per acre.'

"Thus you have the theory, the practice, and the result, of the hogging-off process."

THE RELATION BETWEEN THE PRICES OF CORN AND PORK.

While it is perhaps true, that the bulk of the corn fed to hogs does not give a return of ten pounds of pork, live weight, to the bushel, it *is* established that a bushel of corn *will* make that much, and more, if properly handled, and where it does, the following will serve as a basis for careful calculations :

We present it for what it is worth, and think it may be approximatively correct.

Feeding corn worth 12½ cents per bushel, makes pork costing 1½ cent per pound.

Feeding corn worth 17 cents per bushel, makes pork costing 2 cents per pound.

Feeding corn worth 25 cents per bushel, makes pork costing 2½ cents per pound.

Feeding corn worth from 33 to 40 cents per bushel, makes pork costing 4 cents per pound.

Feeding corn worth 50 cents per bushel, makes pork costing 5 cents per pound.

Or : pork at 5 cents per pound, gross, gives 50 cents per bushel for corn.

At 4 cents per pound, gross, gives from 33 to 40 cents per bushel for corn.

At 2½ to 3 cents per pound, gross, gives from 25 to 30 cents per bushel for corn.

RECORDS AND RECORDING.

Beginning with the organization at Springfield, Illinois, in 1875, of the American Berkshire Association, great attention has been paid in America to recording pedigrees of thoroughbred breeding swine. The value and importance of this are not only quite generally conceded here but also in England, where the British Berkshire Association, following the Yankee example, has already issued ten volumes of herdbooks.

At this writing (January, 1897) there have been issued

fourteen volumes of the American Berkshire Record, containing pedigrees as follows. The table also shows the number of pedigrees in the editor's hands for entry in Volume XV:

	Boars.	Sows.	Total.
Volume I.	235	541	776
" II.	523	1,272	1,795
" III.	480	870	1,350
" IV.	420	735	1,155
" V.	390	780	1,170
" VI.	457	815	1,272
" VII.	693	1,307	2,000
" VIII.	676	1,324	2,000
" IX.	1,155	1,845	3,000
" X.	1,042	1,958	3,000
" XI.	1,167	1,833	3,000
" XII.	1,077	1,923	3,000
" XIII.	1,289	2,711	4,000
" XIV.	1,582	3,418	5,000
" XV.	903	2,118	3,021
Total in fifteen volumes.	12,089	23,450	35,539

The National Berkshire Record, an offshoot of the American, has issued two volumes, containing pedigrees of 535 boars and 1050 sows. In the ten volumes of the British Berkshire Herdbook, so far received, pedigrees have been recorded as below:

	Boars.	Sows.	Total.
Volume I.	156	384	540
" II.	143	297	440
" III.	147	358	505
" IV.	129	335	464
" V.	139	300	439
" VI.	164	359	523
" VII.	170	428	598
" VIII.	144	285	429
" IX.	138	322	460
" X.	145	352	497
Total in ten volumes.	1,475	3,420	4,895

Poland-China breeders have established four separate Records, with different rules, editors and management, instead of coöperating and making one Record and one system of rules, as would seem desirable for any breed. The "Ohio Poland-China Record," having headquarters at Dayton, O., and begun in 1877, has issued already seventeen volumes, with pedigrees of 64,000 animals.

One designated as the "American Poland-China

Record," and thus far published in Iowa, has sent out sixteen volumes since 1878, recording 63,000 pedigrees.

A third, known as the "Central Poland-China Record," had its beginning in Indiana in 1880, and its sixteen issues contain nearly 27,000 pedigrees.

The "Northwestern Poland-China Record," established in Kansas in 1881, but since suspended, issued three volumes.

The fifth and latest established (1886) of these Poland-China Records is named the "Standard," published in Missouri, and its nine volumes are made up of 45,000 pedigrees.

Two Records for Chester Whites have been established —the "Standard" and the "American." The recording done in the "Standard's" five volumes is as follows:

	Boars.	*Sows.*	*Total.*
Volume I.	2,642	2,812	5,454
" II.	245	275	520
" III.	152	260	412
" IV.	224	400	624
" V.	218	412	630
Total in five volumes	3,481	4,159	7,640

The "American"—originally founded as a "Record of Todd's Improved Chester Whites," which were a combination of the Pennsylvania Chester Whites with other white hogs in Ohio, of previously mixed or miscellaneous breeding, since 1865-67—has also published five volumes, made up as here shown:

	Boars.	*Sows.*	*Total.*
Volume I.	190	389	579
" II.	191	363	554
" III.	310	571	881
" IV.	265	408	673
" V.	496	834	1,330
Total in five volumes	1,452	2,565	4,017

The red, or rather sandy, hogs common in America, are by their breeders now designated as Duroc-Jerseys, and two different Records of their pedigrees are now published.

The American Duroc-Jersey Swine Breeders' Association has issued five volumes of its pedigree records, with numbers as below:

	Boars.	*Sows.*	*Total.*
Volume I.	300	1,000	1,300
" II.	400	1,000	1,400
" III.	430	1,000	1,430
" IV.	483	1,000	1,483
" V.	475	1,000	1,475
Total in five volumes	2,088	5,000	7,088

The National Duroc-Jersey Association has issued two volumes of a record containing:

	Boars.	*Sows.*	*Total.*
Volume I.	175	450	625
" II.	450	850	1,300
Total in two volumes	625	1,300	1,925

Two volumes of a Record for the "Victorias," originating in Indiana, have been published, and a third is well towards completion at the time this is written. The following shows the number of pedigrees in each of the two volumes:

	Boars.	*Sows.*	*Total.*
Volume I.	34	69	103
" II.	360	566	926
Total in two volumes	394	635	1,029

An association of Suffolk breeders is expecting to issue the first volume of a Record containing about 350 pedigrees.

The American Essex Association has two volumes with this showing:

	Boars.	*Sows.*	*Total.*
Volume I.	118	233	351
" II.	150	257	407
Total in two volumes	268	490	758

Of the popularity of these various Records, no better evidence is needed than the fact that they are well sustained, and financially prosperous. The prices of the volumes range from $2.00 to $5.00 each, and we believe the fee for recording in any of them is ordinarily $1.00 for each pedigree, except that some of the Record Associations make a special rate of one-half to their shareholders.

STANDARDS OF EXCELLENCE AND SCALE OF POINTS.

Associations of those representing or interested in each of the improved breeds of swine have formulated a standard of excellence or scale of points for their favorites, with about twenty divisions, aggregating one hundred in an animal estimated as perfect in all its points, and it is by these standards that they desire their swine judged at exhibitions.

Below is the standard adopted for Berkshires by the American Berkshire Association, the figures representing the comparative value of each point when perfect:

COLOR—Black, with white on feet, face, tip of tail, and an occasional splash on the arm	4
FACE AND SNOUT—Short; the former fine and well dished, and broad between the eyes	7
EYE—Very clear, rather large, dark hazel or gray	2
EAR—Generally almost erect, but sometimes inclined forward with advancing age; medium size; thin and soft	4
JOWL—Full and heavy, running well back on neck	4
NECK—Short and broad on top	4
HAIR—Fine and soft; medium thickness	3
SKIN—Smooth and pliable	4
SHOULDER—Thick and even, broad on top, and deep through chest	7
BACK—Broad, short and straight; ribs well sprung, coupling close up to hips	8
SIDE—Deep and well let down; straight on bottom lines	6
FLANK—Well back, and low down on leg, making nearly a straight line with lower part of side	5
LOIN—Full and wide	9

HAM—Deep and thick, extending well up on back, and holding thickness well down to hock	10
TAIL—Well set up on back; tapering and not coarse	2
LEGS—Short, straight and strong; set wide apart, with hoofs erect, and capable of holding good weight	5
SYMMETRY—Well proportioned throughout, depending largely on condition	6
CONDITION—In a good, healthy, growing state; not overfed	5
STYLE—Attractive, spirited, indicative of thorough breeding and constitutional vigor	5
TOTAL	100

The following was recommended by the National and has been adopted by the various other Poland-China Associations for that breed:

COLOR—Dark spotted or black	3
HEAD—Small, broad, face slightly dished	5
EARS—Fine and drooping	2
JOWL—Neat and full	2
NECK—Short, full, slightly arched	3
BRISKET—Full	3
SHOULDER—Broad and deep	6
GIRTH AROUND HEART	10
BACK—Straight and broad	7
SIDES—Deep and full	6
RIBS—Well sprung	7
LOIN—Broad and strong	7
BELLY—Wide and straight	4
FLANK—Well let down	3
HAM—Broad, full, and deep	10
TAIL—Tapering, and not coarse	2
LIMBS—Strong, straight, and tapering	7
COAT—Thick and soft	3
ACTION—Prompt, easy and graceful	5
SYMMETRY—Adaptation of the several parts to each other	5
TOTAL	100

The Chester White Association (Todd's) uses the following:

HEAD—Small, broad, slightly dished	7
EAR—Thin, fine, drooping	2
JOWL—Neat and full	4

NECK—Short, full, well arched	3
BRISKET—Full and deep	3
SHOULDER—Broad and deep	6
GIRTH AROUND HEART	9
BACK—Straight and broad	6
SIDES—Deep and full	7
RIBS—Well sprung	6
LOIN—Broad and strong	7
BELLY—Wide and straight	5
FLANK—Well let down	3
HAM—Broad, full, and deep	10
LIMBS—Strong, straight, and neat	6
TAIL—Tapering, and not coarse	2
COAT—Fine and thick	3
COLOR—White	3
SYMMETRY	8
TOTAL	100

The association of breeders of red swine, which they have officially designated and now record as Duroc-Jerseys, has adopted the following scale :

COLOR—Cherry red without other admixture	5
HEAD—Nose fine and short; face slightly dished, wide between eyes	10
EARS—Medium size; not erect nor too drooping	5
CHEEKS—Large, full and well rounded	5
NECK—Short; evenly deep from poll to shoulders	5
SHOULDERS—Broad, smooth and nearly level on top	5
CHEST—Deep; filled level behind shoulders	10
BACK—Broad; straight or slightly arching, carrying even width to hips	10
SIDES—Deep; medium length level between shoulders and hips	10
BELLY—Straight underline; not paunchy	5
HAMS—Large, full, well rounded; extending well to hock joint	10
LEGS—Medium bone; short, straight, well up on toes	5
TAIL—Set medium high; nicely tapering from base	5
HAIR—Fine, soft, straight; moderately thick	5
ACTION—Vigorous, animated, sprightly	5
TOTAL	100

Viewing the accompanying diagram will suggest the

points and method of applying the standard, approximately, to swine of almost any breed :

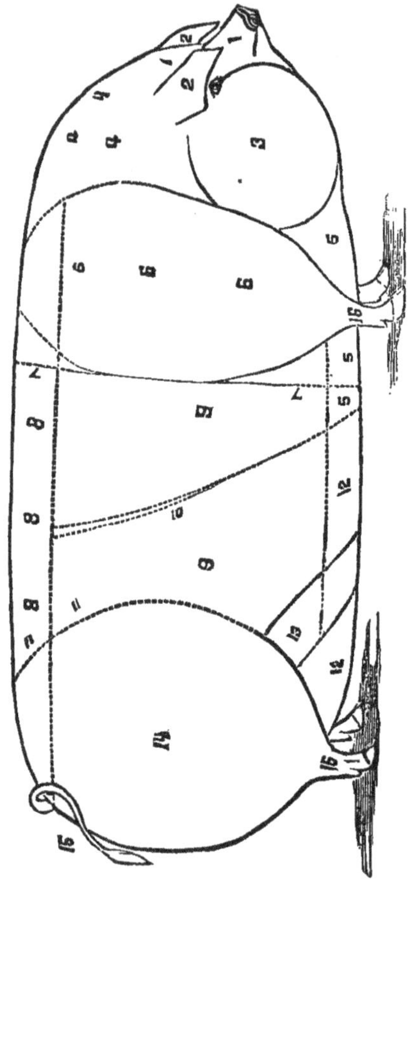

EXPLANATION.—1, Head; 2, Ears; 3, Jowl; 4, Neck; 5, Brisket; 6, Shoulder; 7, Girth around Heart; 8, Back; 9, Sides; 10, Ribs; 11, Loin; 12, Belly; 13, Flank; 14, Ham; 15, Tail; 16, Legs.

COST OF PIG AND PORK.

In recent issues of the *Breeder's Gazette* three different swine-raisers presented statements, each from his own experience, intended to show the cost of young pigs, and also their cost when matured to marketable porkers. The first one, Mr. A. G., makes his figures like this:

"Ten sows, four months old, cost	$100
Interest on the investment, 10 per cent	10
Keep of same one year, 25 bushels of corn each at 30c	75
Keep, interest on cost and shrinkage on boar	10
Extra feed for pigs up to two months old	15
Loss on sows, 20 per cent	20
Cost of pens, $50—interest and repairs, 20 per cent	10
Total	$240

"Allowing fifty pigs from the ten sows, and a loss of thirty per cent up to two months old, and we have thirty-five pigs, costing $140, or $4 each. Allowing a pig at two months to weigh thirty pounds, and nine pounds of pork to a bushel of corn, we will feed him thirty bushels of corn to make him weigh 300 pounds.

"Then we have cost of pig	$4
Thirty bushels of corn at 30 cents	9
Total	$13

"If we add twenty per cent to this to cover the items of labor, taxes, interest and risk after two months old, we have the cost of the 300-pound hog when fit for market, $15.60, or five and a quarter cents a pound, nearly.

"From above calculations pork will cost as follows, nearly:

"Corn at 15 cents, pork will cost	3	cents	per lb.
Corn at 20 cents, pork will cost	3¾	"	"
Corn at 25 cents, pork will cost	4½	"	"
Corn at 30 cents, pork will cost	5¼	"	"
Corn at 35 cents, pork will cost	6	"	""

Swine-raiser number two responds in this way:

"Fortunately, ten sows, the number Mr. A. G. has given in his estimate, is the exact number I kept for several years; but I succeeded in raising to maturity just double his number of pigs to each litter. I usually raise two litters each year, one to come in February and the other in July. My February pigs I fatten the following autumn, and those that come in July are kept through the winter and fed for market the next summer and fall. I think his estimate for the cost of sows—$10 at four months old—is pretty steep for three cent pork. I can always buy sows at that age, suitable for raising pigs, for less than half that amount on a basis of three cent pork, and can raise them cheaper than I can buy. For the sake of comparison I will give the items of expense incurred in raising the little pig:

"Ten sow pigs, four months old	$50.00
Interest on the investment	4 00
Keep of sows 9 months, 15 bushels corn each, 30c	40.50
To pasturing on grass three months	7.50
Interest on cost and keep of boar	8.00
Extra keep of pigs to three months old	30.00
Total	$140.00

"Allowing seventy pigs to ten sows we have the cost of pigs $140, at $2 apiece at three months old. Itemized the account will stand thus:

"Cost of pig at three months	$2.00
Keep for six months, seven bushels corn, at 30c	2.10
Two month's run on clover	50
Fifteen bushels corn to prepare for market	4.50
Total	$9.10

"Thus it will be seen we have the pig ready for market at fourteen months old, and he will weigh 300 pounds—a cost of a fraction over three cents per pound for pork. I have made no allowance for the loss of pigs; but I have only counted one litter to each sow in a year, and given the other litter, which will more than make up for all losses of pigs and sows, and interest on cost of pens; although I have no extra expense for pens, as my hogs have access to the fields the year around with other stock. I regard the manure from the hogs that have the run of the pastures throughout the year as more than equivalent to any pickings that they may get while being fed corn."

Respondent number three presents the results of his experience as follows:

"My experience is that I can buy ten sows, eight months old, at $10 each, and four months later have ten litters averaging seven pigs, or seventy pigs in all. Allowing a loss of thirty per cent up to two months old, at which age I wean them, I have forty-nine pigs to fatten. Now how much have these pigs cost me? I figure it this way:

"Interest on the investment, at 10 per cent	10.00
Keep of ten sows one year	60.00
Keep and interest on boar	10.00
Extra feed on young pigs up to two months	10.00
Loss on sows. (This is counterbalanced by the fact that they will be in pig again.)	
Interest, repairs and labor	20.00
Total	$110.00

"At these figures my young pigs cost me almost exactly $2.25 each. For the next two months I feed these pigs a slop of oats, bran and middlings, costing:

"Feed for two months	$30.00
Labor, etc.	20.00
Total	$50.00

"Now I have forty-nine pigs, four months old, averaging seventy-five pounds, and costing me about $3.25 each. From this time on I feed them corn, twenty-five bushels each, on which they gain 225 pounds, and at a year old they average 300 pounds, and at the following cost:

Cost per head at four months	$3.25
Twenty-five bushels of corn at 20c	5.00
Labor, etc., per head	1.63
Total	$9.88

"Nine dollars and eighty-eight cents is the total cost of my 300-pound hog. I can sell him at our local market at $4.20 (present prices) per 100 pounds, or $12.50 net. I do not feed my brood sows corn in any large quantity, preferring a slop of oats, bran and middlings and an occasional meal of roots. I find this less expensive than corn and I believe less injurious. I pay but twenty cents for corn, and save something in not feeding it to my sows. As I have figured in my estimate the interest and cost of keeping my sows and boar for one year, the second litter will cost only labor and feed for the two months, which amounts to $30 for the forty-nine little pigs, or sixty-one cents each. My first litter cost me $2.25 each at two months old, and this will bring the average cost of all my little pigs, at two months old, down to $1.43. To prove that I am approximately correct, two-months-old pigs can readily be bought in our neighborhood for $2 each."

STOCK YARDS RECEIPTS.

The table on the next page shows the annual and total receipts of hogs at the two greatest live stock markets in the world—the Union Stock Yards, at

Chicago, Illinois, and the Kansas City, Kansas, Stock Yards, since their establishment:

	Chicago, Ill.	*Kansas City, Kan.*
1865, five days	17,764	
1866	961,746	
1867	1,696,738	
1868	1,706,782	
1869	1,661,869	
1870	1,693,158	
1871	2,380,083	41,036
1872	3,252,623	104,639
1873	4,437,750	221,815
1874	4,258,379	212,532
1875	3,912,110	63,350
1876	4,190,006	153,777
1877	4,025,970	192,645
1878	6,339,654	427,777
1879	6,448,330	588,908
1880	7,059,355	676,477
1881	6,474,844	1,014,304
1882	5,817,504	963,036
1883	5,640,625	1,379,401
1884	5,351,967	1,723,586
1885	6,937,535	2,358,718
1886	6,718,761	2,264,484
1887	5,470,852	2,423,262
1888	4,921,712	2,008,984
1889	5,998,526	2,073,910
1890	7,663,829	2,865,171
1891	8,600,805	2,599,109
1892	7,714,435	2,397,477
1893	6,057,278	1,948,373
1894	7,483,228	2,547,077
1895	7,885,283	2,457,697
1896	7,659,472	2,605,575
Total	160,438,972	36,313,120

Chicago, Ill.		*Kansas City, Kas.*	
Largest receipts in one day, Feb. 11, 1895	74,551	Largest receipts in one day, July 30, 1890	26,408
Largest receipts in one week, ending Nov. 20, 1880	300,488	Largest receipts in one week, ending July 31, 1890	155,044
Largest receipts in one month, Nov., 1880	1,111,997	Largest receipts in one month, July, 1890	347,469
Largest receipts in one year, 1891	8,600,805	Largest receipts in one year, 1890	2,865,171

WHEN TO EXPECT THE PIGS.

The period of a sow's gestation being, as a rule, sixteen weeks, the following table is presented as showing exactly when sixteen weeks expires from any day in the year that she may be bred:

January… April……	February… May……	March…… June.. ….	April…… July………	May……. August……	June……. September..	July……. October….	August…. November..	September.. December..	October…. January….	November.. February…	December.. March……
1..22	1..23	1..20	1..21	1..20	1 20	1..20	1..20	1..21	1..20	1..20	1..22
2..23	2..24	2..21	2..22	2..21	2..21	2..21	2..21	2..22	2..21	2..21	2..23
3..24	3..25	3..22	3..23	3..22	3..22	3..22	3..22	3..23	3..22	3..22	3..24
4..25	4..26	4..23	4..24	4 23	4..23	4..23	4..23	4..24	4..23	4..23	4..25
5 26	5..27	5..24	5..25	5..24	5..24	5..24	5..24	5..25	5..24	5..24	5..26
6..27	6..28	6..25	6..26	6..25	6..25	6..25	6..25	6..26	6..25	6..25	6..27
7..28	7..29	7..26	7..27	7..26	7..26	7..26	7..26	7..27	7..26	7..26	7..28
8..29	8..30	8..27	8..28	8..27	8..27	8..27	8..27	8..28	8..27	8..27	8..29
9..30	9..31	9..28	9..29	9. 28	9..28	9..28	9..28	9..29	9..28	9..28	9..30
May	June	10..29	10..30	10..29	10..29	10..29	10..29	10..30	10..29	Mar.	10..31
10.. 1	10.. 1	11..30	11..31	11..30	11..30	11. 30	11..30	11..31	11..30	10.. 1	Apl.
11.. 2	11.. 2	July	Aug.	12..31	Oct.	12..31	Dec.	Jan.	12..31	11.. 2	11.. 1
12.. 3	12.. 3	12.. 1	12.. 1	Sept.	12.. 1	Nov.	12.. 1	12.. 1	Feb.	12.. 3	12.. 2
13.. 4	13.. 4	13.. 2	13.. 2	13.. 1	13.. 2	13.. 1	13.. 2	13.. 2	13.. 1	13.. 4	13.. 3
14.. 5	14.. 5	14 3	14.. 3	14.. 2	14.. 3	14.. 2	14.. 3	14.. 3	14.. 2	14.. 5	14. 4
15.. 6	15.. 6	15.. 4	15.. 4	15.. 3	15.. 4	15.. 3	15.. 4	15.. 4	15.. 3	15.. 6	15.. 5
16.. 7	16.. 7	16.. 5	16.. 5	16.. 4	16.. 5	16.. 4	16.. 5	16.. 5	16.. 4	16.. 7	16.. 6
17.. 8	17.. 8	17.. 6	17.. 6	17.. 5	17.. 6	17.. 5	17.. 6	17.. 6	17.. 5	17.. 8	17.. 7
18.. 9	18.. 9	18.. 7	18.. 7	18.. 6	18.. 7	18.. 6	18.. 7	18.. 7	18.. 6	18.. 9	18 . 8
19..10	19..10	19.. 8	19.. 8	19.. 7	19.. 8	19.. 7	19.. 8	19.. 8	19.. 7	19..10	19.. 9
20..11	20..11	20.. 9	20.. 9	20.. 8	20.. 9	20.. 8	20.. 9	20.. 9	20.. 8	20..11	20..10
21..12	21..12	21..10	21..10	21. 9	21..10	21.. 9	21..10	21..10	21.. 9	21..12	21..11
22..13	22..13	22..11	22. 11	22..10	22..11	22..10	22..11	22..11	22..10	22..13	22..12
23..14	23..14	23..12	23..12	23..11	23..12	23..11	23..12	23..12	23..11	23..14	23..13
24..15	24..15	24..13	24..13	24..12	24..13	24..12	24..13	24 .13	24..12	24..15	24..14
25..16	25..16	25..14	25..14	25..13	25..14	25. 13	25..14	25..14	25 .13	25..16	25..15
26..17	26..17	26..15	26..15	26 14	26..15	26..14	26..15	26..15	26..14	26..17	26 .16
27..18	27..18	27..16	27..16	27..15	27..16	27..15	27..16	27..16	27..15	27..18	27..17
28..19	28..19	28..17	28..17	28..16	28..17	28..16	28..17	28..17	28..16	28..19	28..18
29..20	29..20	29..18	29..18	29..17	29..18	29..17	29..18	29..18	29..17	29..20	29..19
30..21		30..19	30..19	30..18	30..19	30 18	30..19	30..19	30..18	30..21	30..20
31..22		31..20		31..19		31..19	31..20		31..19		31..21

DISEASES OF SWINE.

PRACTICAL INFORMATION AS TO THEIR CAUSES, SYMPTOMS, PREVENTION, AND CURE.

CHAPTER XXIII.

DISEASES OF SWINE AND THEIR TREATMENT.

INTRODUCTORY.

We desire to preface this portion of our volume by saying that we are not a hog doctor, and have but little faith in sick hogs, or in giving them medicines.

A sick hog is, as a rule, very poor property, and he who permits this class of stock to become diseased through negligence or mistreatment, under the impression that "anybody knows enough to doctor a hog," is boldly courting disaster.

The hog has an appetite beyond his powers of digestion; if he is allowed to gorge himself on unsuitable foods, is made to live in filth and mire, from first to last, and is also exposed to burning sun and biting frosts, it can be but small wonder if he becomes the prey of disease.

Prevention, by rational, decent treatment, should be the watch-word; but, if an animal appears ailing, note carefully all the symptoms.

Physicians say that the internal organs of a hog are located much as are those of a man, and that in a majority of cases it will be safe to treat a sick hog, so far as practicable, in the same manner as a sick man should be treated. Medicines ought never to be given without well defined ideas as to what they are expected to accomplish —remembering that "the catalogue of medicine furnishes few, if any *specifics*, that is, medicines that will always *cure* certain diseases."

There are, however, a great number of medicines that appear to be specifics for certain symptoms.

The only really successful way of administering medicine to hogs is, to mix it in their feed or drink, as they are so obstinate and unmanageable that drenching is usually unsatisfactory and always dangerous. If too far gone to eat or drink a little, the case may be considered quite hopeless. They should be made as comfortable as possible, and if they will eat, give them food that is light, and easy to digest, not too much strong medicine, and trust to good care, to time, and to nature, to effect a cure.

The veteran Elmer Baldwin says:

"In winter, I would separate the sick from the herd; give them a good warm sty and access to water, and in summer would turn them where they would have water for both drinking and bathing, with a dense cool shade, and where they would not be disturbed, withhold their feed, and let them take their chances. Such a course I have ever found more successful than any medicine.

"Prevention is better than cure; for a herd of swine properly fed and cared for will seldom be sick, if they are native; their own vital power must cure them; man cannot.

"If they have been improperly fed, until disease has been developed, the best remedy is to change the diet to a proper one.

"If they have been kept in a close pen, exposed to the heat of summer, turn them into a fresh pasture where they can have water, exercise, and shade.

"If they have been kept in a dirty, muddy pen until they have scurf and mange, clean the skin, and give them a clean, comfortable pen to live in. But, better still, give those better conditions before the difficulty occurs. Care for them in advance, both as a matter of duty and profit. And as in morals, the path of duty is the path of happiness and safety, so in the treatment of our domestic animals, generous, kind, and humane treatment brings the most money"

Nothing is more natural than that those who have capital invested in swine should, if disease appears, desire to make some effort to arrest its progress. Appreciating the importance of this, we present here recipes that have been tried, recommended, and endorsed by practical men, who have found them valuable; and we believe them to be more nearly adapted to the wants of swine-breeders than any collection heretofore made.

They are not recommended as infallible, and we would

again impress it upon our readers and fellow-breeders, that the treatment of diseased swine is very uncertain in its results, for when it is so often impossible to ascertain the precise character or location of the ailment, it is indeed difficult to prescribe and administer efficacious remedies. Hence the "ounce of prevention" is all-important.

The information given of the disease or diseases known as Hog Cholera, is unquestionably the best and most thorough that the ablest scientific authorities in the country have as yet arrived at.

ANTHRAX* DISEASES IN SWINE.

The obscure diseases in swine generally—but quite improperly—designated by farmers as "Hog Cholera," have created such fearful ravages in the principal hog-raising districts as to prove the main obstacle to profitable pork production.

There has been witnessed annually, for a generation past, the loss, by epidemic diseases, of millions of dollars worth of swine in this country, at a time of year when they were of maximum value.

It is to be regretted that a scourge so prevalent, carrying disaster and financial ruin to such numbers of our people, has not been made the subject of thorough scientific investigation by a commission, composed of men eminent for their scientific and practical knowledge.

We believe a portion of the appropriation to our National Bureau of Agriculture could, and should, have been used, years ago, to assist in researches to wrest from nature the secret causes of the wide-spread destruction, which, in such numerous instances, makes hog-raising, as a business, so precarious.

If the active pursuit of knowledge so valuable as this does not come within the province of the Department of Agriculture, of State Agricultural Boards and Societies,

* *Anthrax* is the Greek word for carbuncle, or virulent ulcer

and the richly endowed and richly officered Agricultural Colleges, organized ostensibly in the interests of the producing classes, by whom they are largely maintained, we have failed to comprehend their mission, or importance. While such ruinous devastation is abroad in the land, and millions of dollars worth of swine sometimes die in a single month from diseases scarcely understood at all, it is small comfort to the tax-ridden Western farmers to read, in its voluminous reports, that the Department of Agriculture is engaged in investigating the Cranberry-rot in New Jersey, or the Orange-blight in Florida, or that the Massachusetts Agricultural College is making elaborate experiments to test the lifting powers of a *Squash,* which has, at considerable expense, been properly harnessed for that purpose.

No investigation that does not extend through several States, and include thousands of cases, as found under varying and widely different circumstances, and is not made with a liberal and faithfully continued expenditure of time, labor, and some money, can be satisfactory. The necessary expense precludes private investigations from being sufficiently extended, and if properly conducted, the results obtained would be of such general interest that the General Government should lead in the undertaking and bear the expense. Managing our own hogs, on the theory that the "ounce of prevention" was of paramount importance, we have never lost even a single animal by any disease we could call cholera, and as it comprehends conditions and causes regarding which the most learned scientists are as yet groping in comparative darkness, we shall not weary the reader with mere surmises of our own.

Fortunately some two or three of the leading veterinarians in the country have devoted much attention to it, and while none of them claim to have at all solved the mystery in which epidemic diseases are enshrouded, we are able to present, in this and the succeeding chapters, the latest conclusions to which their labors have brought them.

From our standpoint, we consider "hog cholera" as caused by a putrid poison in the blood, induced by unwhole some foods, drink, and surroundings productive of disease, essentially a contagious fever, of which inflammation of the lungs, diarrhœa, vomiting, abscesses, and similar features, are simply complications. Law, and others, do not hesitate to pronounce it as having been known in the Old World, as well as this country, and all authorities encountered by us agree that the unwholesome conditions of life contribute largely to its diffusion, if not its development anew.

Every farmer should realize the necessity of *prevention*, and grasp the fact that the great "cure-all" will never be found, and that trusting to any remedies, specifics, or patent nostrums, is more than likely to result in a disastrous failure, to avert which too much care cannot be taken in securing the best sanitary conditions of life for this class of domestic animals.

Dr. H. J. Detmers, a distinguished veterinarian, who has devoted much research to diseases peculiar to swine in the Mississippi Valley, prepared for and published in the *Rural World*, (St. Louis, April, 1876,) an extended article on Anthrax Diseases in Swine, of which the following is a synopsis:

"Although I have had considerable experience, not only when practising as veterinary surgeon in Europe, but also during the seven years which I have resided in the State of Illinois, I write with some reluctance, because I know that a good deal of what I shall have to say will conflict with some long-cherished notions and prejudices of a great many readers. In the first place, I wish to banish the name of

'HOG CHOLERA,'

which is ill-chosen, entirely without meaning, and leads to confusion, as it naturally conveys the impression that the disease, or diseases so named, are similar to, or identical with the Asiatic cholera, or cholera of men, which is not the case. In fact, what our farmers and swine-breeders are used to call 'hog cholera,' is not a single or separate disease, but rather a group of several kindred diseases, similar to each other in regard to causes, morbid process, contagiousness, and final termination, but differing very much as to symptoms, seat of morbid process, course, and duration. Hence, the proper name,

ANTHRAX DISEASES,

which is understood everywhere, is much preferable to the misnomer 'hog cholera.'

"All anthrax diseases—and those of swine not excepted—make their appearance usually as enzootic diseases. They spread over large districts, and attack a large number of animals of the same kind, and in some cases of different kinds, at once, or in quick succession. Only in comparatively rare cases, one or the other form of anthrax presents itself as a sporadic disease—that is, attacks only a few animals, or remains limited to a farm, a pasture, or a stable, or a yard. This, however, is but natural: in the first place, the presence of the pernicious agencies or influences which constitute the causes is seldom limited to a farm, a pasture, a stable, or a yard, but extends usually over whole districts; and secondly, all anthrax diseases develop a more or less intense contagion, able to communicate the morbid process to other healthy animals, which have not been exposed to the causes, and in severe cases even to men. The morbid process in all anthrax diseases consists in a peculiar decomposition of the blood and of the animal tissues; consequently, everything that is able to introduce or to promote such a decomposition must be considered as a mediate cause.

"CAUSES.

"The causes of the anthrax diseases of swine are essentially the same as those of the anthrax diseases of other domesticated animals. The same proceed, to a great extent, from certain peculiarities of the soil and of the weather, and have their source also—partially at least—in the mode and manner in which the animals are kept. It is possible, according to the scientific investigations and experiments which have been carried on with great zeal during the last decade, that various cryptogamic parasites, the *bacterii*, *vibriones*, and others, found in the blood and in other fluids of anthrax patients, act either directly or indirectly like a ferment upon the blood, effect a decomposition of that fluid, act in that way as a causal agency, or a cause, of the morbid process and its usually fatal termination.

"The experience of our present age, as well as the earliest observations on record, show that anthrax diseases are apt to occur wherever large quantities of stagnant water, surcharged with decomposing vegetable substances, are evaporating. Hence, anthrax diseases may be expected on naturally wet or low land, in a dry season, and on naturally high and dry land, provided the soil is rich in humus, in very wet seasons. The various forms of anthrax, therefore, make their appearance especially as epizootic, or rather enzootic, diseases, in all localities or districts in which the top soil is rich in humus and decomposing vegetable matter, and the subsoil impervious to water, at the end of a wet season, or after an inundation; and in localities or districts in which swamps, sloughs, and pools of stagnant water are numerous and extensive during a hot and dry season, particularly if the animals are compelled to drink foul or stagnant water containing a considerable quantity of decomposing vegetable substances. The water of ponds in which flax has been rotted, must be regarded as extremely dangerous, for this reason.

"Pastures and stubble fields, rich in sulphates, or manured with mineral fertilizers, which effect a more rapid decomposition of the vegetable substances, are also more dangerous than others.

"The weather, too, is not altogether without influence. Weather that is too hot and too sultry for the season of the year, or that is very changeable, (for instance, very warm during the day, and cold at night), seems to promote the outbreak of anthrax diseases. The climate, or the average temperature of a country, is without any consequence, for anthrax makes its appearance as well in the polar regions as in the temperate and in the torrid zones.

"As to the keeping of the animals, it has been observed that sties or pens, full of dung and rotting vegetable substances—clover, weeds, etc.—especially if the latter are wet and exposed to the rays of the sun, have a decidedly bad influence, and are able to act as a cause. Further, certain kinds of food, that contain an abundance of nitrogenous compounds, and are difficult to digest, or very juicy, and of rank and rapid growth, have a great tendency to promote the development of anthrax diseases. As such kinds of food—though some of them are scarcely ever fed to swine—may be named: aftermath clover, the grasses and weeds grown on stubble fields in a wet and warm season, green rye, and green wheat, distillers' mash, moldy hay, spoiled or moldy garden vegetables, musty and moldy grain, and especially grain that contains a great deal of smut. It has been stated time and again, that grasses grown on places or spots where animals diseased with anthrax had died, or had been buried, are able to produce anthrax in living animals. Whether this is true or not, I am unable to decide; I give the statement for what it is worth. Still, it seems that scarcely any one of these more or less injurious kinds of food is able to produce anthrax by itself, but, if acting combined with the influences of evaporating stagnant water, surcharged with decomposing vegetable substances, the same may become very pernicious.

"A great and dangerous predisposition to anthrax diseases is originated, also, by a sudden increase of very nutritious food, causing a rapid improvement of the condition of the animal from poor to good, or from middling good to very good, by accelerating and augmenting rather excessively the organic change of material, or process of wasting and repairing, that is constantly going on in every living organism. If the change of matter is increased too suddenly, or to such an extent that the organs (lymphatics, kidneys, skin, intestines, etc.,) which have the office of disposing of the waste material, and excreting the same, but have been accustomed to only an ordinary quantity of water, cannot absorb and carry off the extraordinary amount that is produced, in consequence of the rapidly-promoted change of matter—a quantity of wasted material, consisting of nitrogenous (urea, for instance,) and carbonaceous compounds, will be retained, and will accumulate in the system, but especially in the blood, where they are apt to become a source of decomposition.

"The predisposing influence of a very rapid growth and improvement in condition, explains why, in every anthrax epizooty, or enzooty, just the most thrifty and fastest improving animals become the victims, and contract, almost invariably, the disease in its most acute and most malignant forms; while the poorest animals in a herd remain either exempted, or take the disease in a less acute, or comparatively mild form. Age and sex seem to be without influence.

"THE CONTAGION.

"A very important source of the spreading of the disease constitutes the contagion. The same is of a fixed, rather than of a volatile nature, and all parts of the animal body (but especially the blood and the fluid products of the morbid process), must be looked upon as its bearers. The vitality of the contagion, and the resistance of the same against external influences, is very great; it is not easily destroyed by exposure to the air, to warmth, cold, moisture, etc. Its intensity, however, is not always the same, but differs according to the form and malignancy of the disease, and the genus of the animal; for it has been repeatedly observed, that contagion in neat cattle, is usually more effective than that developed in horses, or in hogs. It is destroyed most effectually by chemical agencies — for instance, by carbolic acid, chloride of lime, etc.

"The fact that carbolic acid, a most deadly poison to all parasite growth, (vegetable, as well as animal,) destroys also, quicker and more thoroughly than anything else, the efficiency of the contagion developed in anthrax, and in other contagious diseases, may be looked upon as a strong support of the theory which assigns to the cryptogamic parasites, found in the blood and in several other fluids of patients diseased with anthrax, or with any other contagious diseases, a close connection with the contagion.

"The period of incubation (that is, the time which elapses between the exposure to the influence of the contagion and the outbreak of the disease resulting from it), is not always the same, but extends from a few hours to about two weeks. The form of the disease resulting from a contagious infection, is not always identical with the form of anthrax which produced the contagion, but depends upon the seat of the morbid process; and the latter usually localizes itself in the same parts of the body which have been the principal recipients of the contagion.

"Anthrax in swine, as well as in all other domesticated animals, makes its appearance in different forms, which may be divided into two groups—one without any localization of the morbid process, and another one, in which a localization is taking place. The forms belonging to the first group, are characterized by their extremely acute course, and great malignancy. The morbid process affects the whole organism, and has no time to localize itself, but destroys life usually within a few hours, and in some cases even within a few minutes. The forms of anthrax belonging to the second group, are less acute in their course; they last from several hours to several days, and the morbid process, too, is less violent, and has time to effect a localization in one or another part or organ of the animal's body.

"GANGRENOUS ERYSIPELAS.

"Gangrenous, malignant, or contagious erysipelas—St. Anthony's fire, or Wild-fire—must be considered as the most frequent anthrax disease of swine. Its outbreak is usually preceded by some more or less plainly developed precursory symptoms, which, however, often remain unobserved. The animal, a short time before the evident outbreak of the disease, appears to be dull and weak, refuses its food, has an unsteady gait, lies down a great deal, roots in its bedding, and shows a tendency to bury its head (or, if the litter is abundant, its whole body), in the straw. The temperature of the body is changeable, cold shiverings and feverish heat alternate with each other in quick succession ; pulse and respiration are accelerated; the bowels are constipated, or the excrements that are voided are hard and dark-colored; in some cases, the patients make efforts to vomit. In about twelve or twenty-four hours, the symptoms become more characteristic. Red spots, which soon become confluent, make their appearance on the inside of the legs, on the lower part of the abdomen, on the breast, and neck, and soon present an erysipelatous swelling of (at first) a blood-red or crimson, afterwards a purple, and finally (if the termination is to be fatal) a bluish-black color. In some cases, small pustules, with gangrenous, corrosive contents, make their appearance on some parts of the swelled surface; the fever increases in intensity; the mucous membranes present a purple, or lead-gray color; the breathing becomes very laborious; the temperature of the body, at first considerably increased, is much reduced; the hind quarters of the animal become paralyzed, convulsions set in, and the sick animal dies, sometimes within six or twelve hours, but usually on the second or third day after the outbreak of the disease. In those cases in which the animal recovers, the red spots either remain limited, or become less confluent; the fever does not reach so high a degree of intensity, and the other morbid conditions abate, if not before, on the second or third day. Still, some morbid changes, such as partial paralysis in the hind quarters, insufficient appetite (the animals frequently cannot be induced to eat any more than the least amount necessary to keep them alive), defective digestion, etc., often remain, and the recovery is seldom a perfect one.

"The treatment has to be essentially the same as in gangrenous angina. At first an effective emetic, and afterwards calomel, or sulphate of soda, and if the latter is chosen, diluted acids, especially diluted carbolic acid (one part of the crystallized acid to two parts of glycerine, or alcohol, and one hundred parts of water), to be given with extreme care, with a spoon, and in repeated doses, often have a favorable result, provided the treatment is begun before the morbid process has made too much progress. Externally, subcutaneous injections into the swelled parts, of diluted carbolic acid (2½ or 3 parts to 100 of water), have also proved to be of some benefit, and may at least counteract, to a great extent, the septic process.

"MALIGNANT OR GANGRENOUS ANGINA.

"Malignant, or gangrenous, angina is one of the most frequent forms of anthrax, at any rate, more frequent in swine than either apoplectic or gloss anthrax. It usually presents itself as an enzooty, and is therefore often complicated with other forms, especially with malignant erysipelas, so-called St. Anthony's fire, or Wild fire. The morbid process has its principal seat in the throat, in the mucous membranes of the larynx and of the windpipe, and in adjoining parts, but is, in some cases rather concentrated in, or limited to, a certain part—the larynx, for instance—and in other cases more diffused. Consequently, some patients present more outside swelling, or show greater distress and difficulty of breathing than others, although the disease is the same.

"The principal symptoms, though not all of them are alike conspicuous in every patient, consist in wheezing and laborious breathing, hoarse grunting, great heat, and dryness of the snout, swelling of the tongue, a brown-red color of the mucous membranes of the mouth, difficulty in swallowing the food, and attempts to vomit. In the larynx region, and along the windpipe, appears a hot, hard, and painful swelling, which not seldom extends downward and backward to the forelegs, or even to the lower surface of the chest and abdomen. The swelled parts present, at first, a saturated red or crimson, afterwards, often, a reddish lead-gray, and finally a purple color, and an œdematous character. The fever is usually very high; the sick animals breathe with increasing difficulty, and either lie down, or sit on their haunches, like a dog. Finally, the difficulty of breathing becomes so great, that desperate attempts have to be made to catch a little air by opening the mouth, and protruding the livid-colored and swelled tongue. The mucous membrane of the mouth, at first red-brown, changes its color to lead-gray; the temperature of the body, at first considerably higher than in a healthy animal, decreases below the normal degree, and the patients either die of suffocation, or in consequence of the spreading gangrene, within one or two days. In those cases in which the morbid process has concentrated itself in the larynx, the patients suffocate a great deal sooner, and die, sometimes, within an hour after the appearance of the morbid symptoms.

"If the disease does not terminate in death, which is but seldom the case, unless the patients are subjected to a rational treatment during the very first stages of the disease, the morbid symptoms are gradually reduced. In such a case, the respiration becomes freer and less laborious; the wheezing disappears; the difficulty in swallowing food and water abates, and the external swelling ceases to spread, and finally decreases gradually in size. Malignant angina, as well as other forms of anthrax, has either an idiopathic origin, or is the consequence of an infection brought about, in most cases, by eating meat, blood, etc., of animals that have died of anthrax.

"A treatment, to be of any avail, must be instituted during the very first stages of the disease. It is best to commence by giving a good emetic, consisting of two to twenty grains (according to the age and size of the patient) of powdered White Hellebore (*Veratrum album*), or of Tartar Emetic. The former, however, is more reliable, and therefore to be preferred. Both medicines must be given, either with a little milk—if the patient will take them voluntarily—or, mixed with a pinch of flour and a little water, or a piece of boiled potato, in form of pills—if force is necessary, but under no circumstances in the shape of a drench. If the animal should not vomit freely within twenty minutes, the dose has to be repeated. Afterwards, the so-called antiphlogistic salts—sulphate of soda, sulphate of potash, sulphate of magnesia, saltpetre, or calomel, may be given to some advantage. Diluted acids, vegetable as well as mineral, but especially diluted carbolic acid (1 to 100 of water), and subcutaneous injections of diluted carbolic acid (2½ or 3 parts of the acid, 5 parts of glycerine, and 95 parts of water), made into the swelled parts at various places, have been used to advantage, and have given, in many cases, at least, much better satisfaction than anything else. Some authors have advised to draw setons or rowels, to fix the swelled parts with a red-hot iron, or to apply cold water douches, but if the nature of the disease is taken into consideration, it is difficult to see what good such remedies can do. Blood-letting, too, has been recommended, but if resorted to, it must be done during the very first, or incipient, stage of the disease, otherwise it will only accelerate the fatal termination.

"As preventive remedies, diluted acid, sour buttermilk, unripe sour apples, once a week a dose of sulphate of soda, and especially, now and then, a little carbolic acid in the water for drinking, have proved of some value.

"ANTHRAX CARBUNCLE, OR WHITE BRISTLE.

"Real anthrax carbuncle is of comparatively rare occurrence in hogs. Its outbreak is always attended with very severe fever, and the carbunculous swelling usually makes its appearance on the neck, in close proximity to the larynx, and is extremely painful. The bristles, or hair, on such a carbuncle, become bleached, hard, and brittle, and stand on end, therefore the name "white bristle." Finally, great difficulty of breathing, groaning, gnashing and grating of the teeth, and convulsions, constitute the last symptoms and the precursors of death, which ensues usually within a few days.

"The local treatment consists in destroying, or cauterizing, the carbuncles as soon as possible, by means of a red-hot iron, or with a concentrated acid. The general treatment has to be the same as in malignant angina.

"APOPLECTIC ANTHRAX.

"The apoplectic form of anthrax, the most acute of all, is not so frequent in hogs as in cattle and sheep, but wherever it occurs, it usually terminates within so short a time, that the owner of the smitten animals will either find them dead, or will just come in time to see them break down and die, before he even suspected them of being sick. Death is almost instantaneous, and treatment, therefore, is out of the question. Some twelve or fourteen years ago, one of my own pigs, a nice, thrifty animal of common stock, died of this form of anthrax. It stepped back from the trough, turned around, squealed, tumbled down, and died in less than half a minute. In some—though still rarer—cases the termination is not quite so rapid; the diseased animals manifest sickness, by showing symptoms of distress; their gait becomes unsteady and swaggering; the visible mucous membranes appear very much reddened; the temperature of the body changes from feverish heat to cold shiverings, which follow each other in rapid succession. After this stage, the sick animals frequently vomit a bloody or discolored fluid, and usually die very soon, under convulsions. In some cases, carbuncles or erysipelatous swellings make their appearance a short time before death, indicating a tendency of the morbid process to localize itself.

"THE MOUTH, GUM, OR GLOSS ANTHRAX,

or malignant pustule of hogs, is one of the most acute forms of the second group, and a comparatively rare disease.

"Restlessness, loss of appetite, a distressful and staring expression of the eyes, abnormal heat in the mucous membranes of the mouth, gnashing the teeth, and slavering, constitute the first morbid symptoms, and the first indications of the presence of disease and high fever. Very soon, however, (at any rate within an hour or two), one or more, but seldom many, pustules, each the size of a pea, or a bean, make their appearance on the tongue, the gums, and in other parts of the mouth. These pustules, surrounded at their base by an erysipelatous swelling, are first yellowish-white, but change their color very soon to brown, and finally to black, according to the changes which their fluid contents are undergoing. The fever, at the same time, has become very severe. These pustules, if not early enough removed and destroyed, together with their contents, will soon break and discharge their gangrenous fluid, which will cause mortification in every tissue with which it comes in contact. In such a case the animal will die, usually within a few hours, but at any rate within a few days. As a general rule in this, as well as all other forms of anthrax, the better the condition of the patient, the sooner does it terminate in death. The treatment, on account of the very acute course, and of the peculiar seat of the disease, is difficult. The pustules have to be opened, and emptied of their contents, by means of a small spoon with somewhat sharp or thin edges, (one made of tin will answer best), and the remaining sores have to be cauterized, with either sulphuric, hydro-chloric, nitric, or carbolic acid. The opening and destroying of the pustules, and the application of the acid, are attended with some danger to the operator, unless he is very careful not to soil his hands with the contents of the pustules. A person with sores on his hands should never undertake it. The whole operation, however, is useless, unless the pustules are opened in a very dexterous manner, and their contents removed at once, so as to prevent the animal from swallowing them. The general treatment has to be the same as that of the foregoing forms of anthrax.

"PREVENTION

"As to prevention, really not much remains to be said. Removing the causes, and, as the disease is contagious, separating the healthy animals from the sick ones, and destroying the contagion wherever it exists, by means of crude carbolic acid or with chloride of lime—constitute the principal and most important measures of prevention. Besides this, care must be taken, wherever it is intended to improve the condition of an animal, to do so gradually—to feed regularly at all times, and give nothing but what is healthy and sound. That pure, clean water for drinking, is absolutely necessary, and that troughs, sties, or pens, and yards, have to be kept as clean and dry as possible—need to be specially mentioned. In those sections of the country, in which the natural condition of the soil is such as to invite a development of anthrax diseases, where, in other words, the top soil consists of a rich humus, and the subsoil of an impervious clay, or where sloughs and swamps are extensive and numerous, or where the country is subject to inundations—proper draining, thorough cultivation, drying of the swamps and wet places, and building dykes or levees, or digging canals, to prevent the inundations, constitute the only preventives that can be applied. Medicines, in such cases, are of no avail; they can be used to advantage only where it becomes necessary to assist the organism in ejecting waste material. Hence, the feeding of copperas, charcoal, sulphur, saltpetre, salt, ashes, and all the hundred and one other things, that have been recommended, is perfectly useless, if not injurious, and has never prevented a solitary case of anthrax, or so-called hog cholera. I am sure my own Berkshires are as healthy and thrifty animals as can be found anywhere, and they never receive anything of that kind; but they are regularly fed, have good sties, spacious yards, and, what is most important, plenty of pure spring water to drink, and to take a bath in, whenever they feel like it."

CHAPTER XXIV.

THE SO-CALLED "HOG CHOLERA."

THE REPORT OF DR. H. J. DETMERS.

During the year 1875, and for the greater part of 1876, there prevailed, in Missouri, a disease among swine, to an alarming extent, which was called by the farmers "hog cholera." The same disease, or one closely resembling it, was exceedingly destructive in Illinois, and other hog-producing States. The Missouri State Board of Agriculture, recognizing the fact that a disease must be understood before proper curative, or even preventive means could be employed, assigned to Dr. H. J. Detmers, Professor of Veterinary Science in the State Agricultural College, the duty of investigating the disease in its various forms and in all its stages. His examinations were made in different parts of the State, on both living and dead animals, and animals with the disease in various degrees of development were killed, to allow of post-mortem examinations, careful inspections were made of localities in which the disease was most prevalent, etc. The results of his labors are embodied in a Report to the Board, dated Sept. 8, 1876. This Report, with the exception of a few unimportant paragraphs, is here given :

"THE NATURE OF THE DISEASE.

"The morbid process presents itself in a majority of cases as a *catarrhal rheumatic*, and in others as a *gastric rheumatic or billious rheumatic affection*, and exhibited always more or less plainly, a decidedly typhoid character. As a catarrhal rheumatic affection it has its principal seat in the mucous membranes of the respiratory passages, in the substance of the lungs, in the *pulmonal pleura* or serous membrane coating the external surface of the lobes of the lungs, in the *costal pleura* or serous lining of the internal surface of the chest, in the *diaphragm*, and in the *pericardium*, or serous bag enveloping the heart. As a gastric-rheumatic affection, the principal seat of the disease is found in the abdominal cavity, but especially in the liver, in the spleen or milt, in the large and small intestines, in the kidneys and ureters, and in the *peritoneum* or serous membrane lining the interior surface of the abdominal cavity, and constituting the external coat of most of the organs situated in that part of the body. Hence, the name Hog Cholera is an ill-chosen one; it tends to convey the idea that the disease in question is similar to, or identical with, the cholera of men, which is not the case; therefore the application 'hog cholera,' which has already led to a great many mistakes in regard to treatment and measures of prevention, should be abolished at once, and a more appropriate name should take its place. As such a one I wish to propose '*Epizootic Influenza of Swine*,' for two reasons: First, the disease in question bears, in all its morbid features, and especially in the diversity of its forms, produced by the differences in the seat of the morbid process, a striking resemblance to the yet well-remembered epizootic influenza of horses, which swept the whole country a few years ago from the Atlantic to the Pacific; second, I admit it might be more convenient to select a name derived from a conspicuous and characteristic symptom, or from an important and constant morbid change—pleuro-pneumonia of swine, for instance—if the main seat of the morbid process was always in the respiratory organs, or invariably the same in every patient. But as this is not the case, as the seat of the disease is found not only in the respiratory apparatus, but also, in a large number of cases, in the parts and organs connected with the digestive process, and, in some cases, even in the centres of the nervous system, a name had to be chosen that is comprehensive enough in its meanings to cover all the different forms under which the disease is able to make its appearance, and, at the same time, sufficiently distinct to prevent any diagnostic confusion. As such a name I cannot think of any that would answer better than that of Epizootic Influenza of Swine, which, therefore, I recommend for a general adoption.

"SYMPTOMS AND MORBID CHANGES.

"As the morbid process has its seat in various organs or parts of the body, the disease presents itself in different forms, and manifests its presence by different symptoms, so that, at any rate, besides other complications, two principal, and two subordinate, forms or varieties must be discriminated.

1. *The Catarrhal Rheumatic Forms.*—This is the most frequent of the two principal forms. The morbid process has its main seat in the respiratory organs; the disease presents the features of a respiratory disorder, and either the catarrhal or the rheumatic character predominates, or both are equally developed. If the latter is the case, the whole respiratory apparatus may be found diseased. If the catarrhal character is the one that is most developed, the principal seat of the disease will be found in the larynx, in the windpipe, in the bronchial tubes, and, to a larger or smaller extent, in the substance of the lungs; and if the rheumatic form is the predominating one, the principal morbid changes occur in the serous membranes of the chest, (the *costal* and *pulmonal pleura* and the *pericardium*), and also, to some extent, in the tissue of the lungs. In most cases, however, the catarrhal and the rheumatic character are blended with each other, and the respiratory passages, the tissue of the lungs, and the serous membranes, or parts of them, are more or less diseased.

"Animals afflicted with the catarrhal rheumatic form indicate the presence of the disease by a short, more or less hoarse, hacking cough—generally one of the first symptoms—by difficulty of breathing, a panting or drawing motion of the flanks at each breath, by holding the head in a peculiar, stretched, and somewhat drooping position, by a slow and undecided gait, a peculiar hoarseness when caused to squeal, etc. The attending fever is severe enough to announce its presence by unmistakable symptoms, such as accelerated pulsation, changeable temperature, etc. Some of the sick animals show at the beginning of the disease a tendency to vomit, and have diarrhœa, while others are more or less constipated from the first, and remain constipated till the disease is ready to terminate in death. If the catarrhal character is the most prevailing, but especially if the morbid process has developed itself principally in the throat and in the windpipe, more or less swelling (quinsy) will make its appearance.

"At the post mortem examination some important morbid changes will invariably be found in the lungs. Portions of the same have become impervious to air by being gorged with exudation. The diseased tissue has lost its spongy feature, has become heavier, and more solid, similar in appearance and consistency to a piece of liver —a condition called *hepatization*. In some cases the diseased or hepatized parts of the lungs present a uniform red or reddish-brown color, and indicate that the exudation has been produced, and been deposited in the tissue of all the diseased lobules, at the same time, or without interruption. In other cases, the single lobules in the diseased portions of the lungs present different colors; some are red, some brown, and others gray or yellowish-gray, which gives the whole hepatized part a somewhat marbled appearance, and shows that the exudation has been produced and been deposited at different periods. The gray hepatization, which is the oldest, and the brown, which comes next in age, contain frequently a few tubercles, or even here and there a small ulcer interspersed. Otherwise neither ulceration nor suppuration has been observed. Important morbid changes are usually found also in the serous membranes of the thorax. The same consist in a more or less firm coalescence between parts of the pulmonal pleura and the corresponding parts of the costal pleura, and in an accumulation of a larger or smaller quantity of straw-colored water or serum in the chest. In other cases, those in which the rheumatic character has been predominating, the morbid products of the diseased serous membranes are frequently very copious; the adhesion between the pulmonal and costal pleura, or between the external surface of the lungs and the internal surface of the walls of the thorax, is usually very extensive; and in some cases parts of the posterior surface of one or both lungs are found firmly united with the corresponding parts of the diaphragm or membraneous partition which separates the chest from the abdominal cavity. The quantity of serous exudation, or straw-colored water deposited in the chest is often very large, and the pericardium, too, contains in most cases a larger or smaller quantity, sometimes enough to interfere seriously with the functions of the heart, and to constitute thereby the immediate cause of death. The blood is found to be thin and watery in every case, and coagulates rapidly to a uniform, but somewhat pale-red clot and of loose texture. Its quantity is always very small.

"2. *The Gastric Rheumatic Form.*—This form presents itself not quite so often as the catarrhal rheumatic, but is fully as malignant, and constitutes the second main form which the disease is found to assume. The morbid process has its principal seat, and produces the most important morbid changes, in some of the organs situated in the abdominal cavity, but especially in the liver, in the spleen or milt, in the kidneys, the ureters, in the intestines or guts, and almost invariably in the peritoneum or serous membrane, which lines the interior surface of the abdominal cavity, and constitutes the external coat of nearly every intestine.

"The symptoms which present themselves while the animal is living, differ not very essentially from those observed in the catarrhal rheumatic form. The short, hacking cough, characteristic of the latter, is more or less wanting; the difficulty of breathing is less plain; the weakness in the hind quarters, and the staggering or unsteady gait, observed only in limited degrees in the catarrhal rheumatic form, is more conspicuous, and the fever is fully as high in one form as in the other.

"In severe cases, the affected animals arch their backs, or rather the lumbal portion of the same to a very high degree, so that the outline of the back resembles somewhat the shape of an ∞. I observed this especially in those cases in which the morbid process has established itself in the kidneys and in the ureters, and in which a large quantity of serous exudation, or straw-colored water, had accumulated in the abdominal cavity.

"Animals affected with the gastric form, show usually more or less costiveness of the bowels. The dung is of the consistency of shoemaker's wax, and is voided in small, irregular-shaped balls, which are usually coated with a layer of grayish or discolored mucus. Still, if the disease is near its fatal termination, the constipation, in many cases, gives way to a profuse and fetid diarrhœa, which may be looked upon, in every instance, as a very fatal sign, and a forerunner of death.

"The principal morbid changes, as I have found them, are as follows: 1. Degeneration of the liver, brought about by a copious exudation infiltrated into the tissue of that organ. Such a degeneration, although not a constant morbid change, is found quite often. In some, not very frequent cases, a few tubercles, and in others, still less frequent, even a few very small abscesses, have been found imbedded in the diseased substance of the liver. 2. Morbid enlargement of the spleen or milt. I found this change in nearly every case. In some cases, the enlargement was not very conspicuous, but in others the spleen was more than three times its natural size, was perfectly gorged with blood, presented a dark black-brown color, and was so soft that very slight pressure with a finger was sufficient to sever its tissue. 3. In quite a large number of them I found one or both kidneys diseased, enlarged, and presenting an inflamed appearance. In one case, both kidneys and both ureters exhibited a high degree of inflammation, and considerable gangrenous destruction. The latter, however, was probably not a consequence of the disease; the animal had been drenched repeatedly with oil of turpentine, and was the only one in which I found any gangrene. In another animal, which, by the way, was already convalescent, and was killed by bleeding, I found one kidney enlarged to three times its natural size, its pelvis very much distended, and its funnel-shaped ureter dilated to such an extent, where it proceeds from the kidney, as to present a diameter nearly one inch and a half. The walls of the ureter were very thick and callous, especially at the anterior, funnel-shaped end, and the latter contained in its interior a semi-solid, fibrous substance, which occupied the whole cavity, and extended even into the kidney. 4. In some cases, I found the membranes of the intestines, or guts, but especially those of the jejunum or small intestine, of the cœcum and colon, or larger intestines, and also the rectum, in a more or less inflamed and degenerated condition. In two cases, a whole convolution of the jejunum had united to an almost solid bunch. On opening the latter, I found, in each case, all three membranes, but particularly the external or serous membrane, and the internal or mucous membrane, very much swelled and degenerated, the passage nearly closed, and in a small cavity in the centre of the bunch, one or two large round worms (*Echinorhynchus gigas*) imbedded. In another case I found, besides other morbid changes, a few round worms in the stomach, and in the mucous membrane of the guts or intestines, a large number of callous scars, such as are usually left behind where the gigantic *Echinorhynchus*, or hook-headed worm, had been fastening itself. These three cases just mentioned, are the only ones in which I have found any entozoa, or worms, in the digestive canal. 5. In almost every case, I found larger or smaller portions of the peritoneum or serous membrane which lines the inner surface of the walls of the abdominal cavity, and the external surface of nearly every intestine, swelled and more or less inflamed, and mobility changed. In some cases, even a coalescence between parts of the intestines, especially the jejunum and rectum, and the walls of the abdominal cavity had been effected; in case, a part of the jejunum had become firmly united to the lower border of the right lobe of the liver, and in another the whole rectum adhered so firmly to the upper wall of the pelvis and of the posterior part of the abdominal cavity that it required the use of a knife to affect a separation. 6. I found in every animal that had been affected with the gastric rheumatic form of the disease, a larger or smaller quantity of the straw-colored water or serum, and small lumps and flakes of coagulated fibrine in the abdominal cavity; in some cases, the quantity was quite a large one, and in others the quantity was comparatively small.

"Two cases must be considered as subordinate forms, in which either one of the principal forms—the catarrhal rheumatic and gastric rheumatic—is essentially modified by being complicated with an affection of the brain and its membranes, or with a serious disorder of the lymphatic system. Hence, two subordinate forms have to be added.

"The perspiration—perceptible and imperceptible perspiration—can be interrupted, or in other words, the skin can be disqualified to perform its functions by several means; for instance, by a disturbance or partial interruption of the circulation of the blood in its capillary vessels, by congestion, inflammation or degeneration of its tissue, or of a part of its tissue, by a closing of its pores by mechanical means, etc. This granted, it remains to ascertain, if those hogs and pigs which have been, or which are yet, affected with the epizootic influenza of swine (erroneously hog cholera), have been subjected to one or more of those just named influences, or agencies, able to cause an interruption or partial cessation of the perspiration. Taking these facts just as they have presented themselves, that question must be answered in the affirmative. My investigations and my inquiries have convinced me that in all those hogs or pigs which have suffered from, or died of, that disease, one or more of those influences or agencies have been at work, as I shall try to show.

"1. All animals affected with that disease—at any rate, all those which I have seen, and I have seen a very large number—were exceedingly lousy. Lice irritate the skin, keeping it in a semi-inflamed condition, cause swelling, and finally a gradual degeneration of its external layer, and constitute, therefore, beyond a doubt, a cause disturbing to some extent the normal perspiration.

"2. All the hogs and pigs which have contracted the disease, have been exposed, night and day, to all the sudden changes of temperature and weather so frequent in our Western States. Some of the animals have been kept in small, wet, and dirty yards, or inclosures, without a roof to protect them; they had to suffer during the day from the rays of the sun, and from the heat which naturally accumulated in a small space, or lot, walled in by a tight fence, and is constantly increased by the wet manure and other organic substances. During the night, the same animals were exposed to the chilling influence of the cold night air, and frequently very heavy dews, not to mention the effects of severe rains and thunder storms. Further, after each heavy rain, the animals thus kept had a chance to get their whole body covered with mud, and the pores of their skin thoroughly closed, but an opportunity to get rid of the mud by taking a bath in clean water, was never given. Such influences, evidently, are very apt to cause irregularities in the circulation of their blood in the capillary vessels of the skin, and, in consequence, an interruption of the perspiration. Other animals have been kept in comparatively large herds, and have been allowed to run at large in the barnyard, in a so-called hog-lot, in the woods, etc. These, too, were exposed more or less to the burning rays of the sun during the day, but during the night, the same, in most cases, found shelter under a corn-crib, under an old stable, or an old barn, or, at any rate, in the closest and dirtiest places, where they lacked room, and where they were often crowded on top of each other when retiring to sleep. As a consequence, the animals became heated and perspiring; and took cold and became chilled when they rose in the morning from this common lair. A sudden cooling, however, or a sudden reduction of temperature of the surface of the body, is apt to effect a contraction of the capillary vessels of the skin, hence diminished supply of blood, and, in consequence, a decrease or partial interruption of the functions of the skin. The animals, thus suddenly cooled by the cool morning air and the wet dew, become, in the course of the forenoon, again exposed to the rays of the sun and the heat of the day, which induces them to go into the first pool of water —if one was accessible—to take a bath. This is all right and well enough, because, in the summer, a hog should have access to water, and an opportunity to take a bath as often as it desires. In all those places, however, in which the disease has made its appearance. I have found the water to which the hog had access, almost invariably so shallow, and of such a limited quantity, that the bathing and wallowing of one of a few animals was sufficient to convert the same into a sticky, semi-fluid mud. Consequently, if the herd was a large one, only a few animals—and these invariably the stronger and most active ones—had now and then a chance to find clean water, and to reap real benefit from taking a bath. All others, but especially the younger and smaller animals (shotes), were compelled to wait till the first comers were through with their bathing, and had changed the water to mud ; the former, therefore, had scarcely ever an opportunity to clean themselves from the mud of the preceding day, and to open the pores of the skin by taking a bath in clean water. If they wish to take a little cooling, they have to be satisfied with a mud-bath, and as every new bath is a mud-bath again, the pores of the skin, as a consequence, instead of being opened, will become closed more and more effectually from day to day, until finally the perspiration will be thoroughly interrupted, and the result, disease, will make its appearance. It is different if the herd is a small one, for then nearly every animal will have, sometimes, a chance to open the pores of its skin by a bath in tolerably clean water, and the perspiration will not be seriously interrupted. That these directions must be correct, can be proved by my observations, which show that in almost every large herd, nearly all the younger and weaker animals (shotes), have become a prey to the disease, while the large and stronger, or most active animals, which are usually the first ones to go to the water in the morning, when the same is yet tolerably clean, and which usually secure at night the best places in the common lair, have either remained exempt, or have had the disease in a milder form, and have mostly recovered. Finally, small herds have either suffered fewer losses, have been less severely attacked, or have remained exempt altogether.

"2. *Agencies which interfere directly with the process of breathing, and foreign substances which enter the respiratory passages.* These, too, as already indicated, are of a different character. When I first commenced my investigation, it struck me that all these swine —pigs, shotes, and grown hogs, of every age and description— which run at large in the streets and thoroughfares of Kansas City, Westport, Independence, Lexington, and other places, and lead the most independent life possible, but do not congregate, go home in the evening, and belong to parties who own but one, two, or may be three animals, as also all those swine which are kept by themselves, either one by one, or only a few together, and, finally, all those which are kept in comparatively small herds, in pastures, orchards, or woods, coated everywhere with grass, and perfectly destitute of dusty, bare ground, and of old manure heaps, are, remain, and have been, with rare exceptions, perfectly healthy. I say, with rare exceptions, for it has been reported to me that a few of these swine running at large in the streets have died, but I have not been able to ascertain with certainty the causes of their death. On the other hand, all those animals which have been kept in yards, pastures, or fields, etc., which consist partially or wholly of bare, dusty ground, or which contain heaps and accumulations of old manure, have suffered, and are suffering severely, and the more so the larger the herd, and the worse the dust of soil and manure. In large herds, composed of 100 head or more, the mortality has been as high as from 70 to 90 per cent; in smaller herds, the same has been from 25 to 60 per cent, and where only a few animals have been kept together, and consequently each animal was compelled to inhale only the dust kicked up by itself, and occasionally, by one or two others, the mortality has been very low, has seldom exceeded 10 per cent, or no fatal cases have occurred at all. Further, in all those cases, in which the hogs or pigs have been compelled to inhale, with each breath, a large quantity of soil and manure, ground to a fine powder by the rays of the sun, and by heat, rain, wind, tramping, and rooting, all the *post mortem* examinations—and I have made a large number during the last four weeks—have revealed as principal morbid changes a morbid affection of the eyes, inflammation of the respiratory passages (throat, wind-pipe, bronchial tubes), hepatization of the lungs in various stages of development, and, in some cases, even some tubercles, or a few small abscesses in the pulmonal tissue, while the serous membrane (pulmonal and costal pleura, pericardium, and peritoneum) presented themselves in a comparatively healthy condition, except in those cases in which the causes described under 1 had acted with those under discussion.

"If these facts just related are duly taken into consideration, scarcely any doubt can remain that the constant inhalation of powdered soil and manure constitutes one of the principal causes of the epizootic influenza of swine.

"As another noxious influence, injuring the organs of respiration, may be considered the effluvia emanating from old, decomposing manure heaps, or farm accumulations of filth, and dirt in pig-sties or hog-yards; but as these are only of subordinate importance, I do not deem it necessasy to enter into further details.

"3. *The auxiliary, or aggravating, and predisposing causes.* As such, I have to consider all the injurious agencies, or noxious influences, which are calculated to promote or to develop the typhoid character of the disease, to weaken the constitution of the animal, or to produce a predisposition. As belonging to this class, I have to mention first, as having a very injurious effect upon the animal system, an impure, foul, or filthy condition of the water for drinking; and secondly, the filth and manure which the animals are obliged to consume with their food. On most farms, the swine are fed with corn in the ear, which, on a great many farms, is thrown to them with great carelessness, in the very filthiest and dirtiest places, so that scarcely a kernel of corn can be picked up free from dirt or manure. That such a wholesale consumption of dirt and excrements must finally undermine the constitution of even the healthiest and most vigorous animal, and must give to any disease that may happen to affect the same some typhoid character, is too evident to need much explanation.

"3. *The Cerebro-Rheumatic Form.*—The same, though always blended with, and in a certain degree subordinate to, one of the two principal forms, has been observed in a large number of sick animals. The latter, besides exhibiting all the symptoms of one or another of the principal (catarrhal-rheumatic or bilious-rheumatic) forms, show also plain indications of morbid affection of the brain. These indications consist principally in partial or perfect blindness, a very staggering gait, and aimless movements in general.

"On opening the skull, I found, invariably, more or less swelling in the membranes enveloping the brain, a larger or smaller quantity of serum deposited inside of the hard membrane (*dura mater*), the substance of the brain more or less softened, and the small cavities or ventricles of the latter organ filled with serum. The other morbid changes found at the *post mortem* examinations are the same that have been described under the head of their respective form.

"4. *The Lymphatic-Rheumatic Form.*—The same, too, has been observed quite often, but always as a complication of one of the principal forms, described under 1 and 2. The whole morbid process presents a somewhat scrofulous character. The lymphatic system is plainly affected; tumors and ulcers showing a scrofulous character, are found in various parts of the body, but especially on the gums. Hence there can be no doubt that such cases, although complicated and blended invariably to such an extent with one or another of the main or principal forms, as to make it impossible to draw distinct lines, have to be looked upon as a subordinate form, with a lymphatic character.

"I have been informed repeatedly, by reliable persons, that in some of the sick animals cutaneous eruptions have constituted one of the most conspicuous symptoms of the disease. If this is a fact, it is possible that yet a fifth (erysipelatous) form has been added. Still, I have had no chance to examine such a patient, notwithstanding that I have seen a large number of sick animals, exceeding, I should judge, one thousand; I am, therefore, not prepared to decide whether the cutaneous eruption is a product of the same morbid process which is at the bottom of the other morbid changes, or whether the same is an independent disease, and merely an accidental complication.

"It is probably not necessary to mention that the morbid changes which have been described as the products or attendants of a certain form, are but seldom found as a total in one and the same animal, as one or more of them are usually missing, or but little developed. Neither will it be essential to state that even the two principal forms of epizootic influenza of swine—leaving the subordinate forms out of consideration—are scarcely ever observed entirely independent of each other, or without being complicated in the least with any other form; that, on the contrary, the gastric rheumatic and the catarrhal rheumatic are, in many instances, blended and complicated with each other to such an extent as to make it impossible to decide which one has to be considered as the most predominating. In such cases, the symptoms, too, are blended with each other, and morbid changes, frequently of equal importance, are found in both large cavities in the chest and in the abdomen. These facts are easily understood by any one who is at all familiar with pathology and with morbid anatomy. The main or fundamental character of epizootic influenza of swine is always rheumatic, and principal seat is the system of the serous membranes, abounding in every large cavity of the animal body. Serous membranes not only line the interior of those cavities, but constitute, also, the external coat of nearly every internal organ. Hence it is but natural that such disease should localize in many different parts of the animal organism, to produce, in consequence, different morbid symptoms, and to cause different forms of disease. It is true, that, in some cases, the disease exhibits a prevailing catarrhal character; but if it is taken into consideration that the causes of rheumatic affection and of catarrhal diseases are often essentially the same, and that the seat or character of a disorder depend, frequently, upon an individual predisposition of the animal, a further explanation will not be needed.

"THE CAUSES.

"To ascertain the causes has been my principal object. It was, therefore, necessary to observe a large number of cases, and to investigate the disease in different localities. This I have done, and have come to the conclusion that some of the causes—and I think I am not mistaken if I say the most important ones—are of such a nature as to admit removal, notwithstanding that they are diverse and numerous, and have their source, to a certain extent, in the manner of farming and stock raising in the West. Although I will not deny the possibility of an existence of certain agencies of a so-called cosmic or telluric character, calculated to act as a cause or to contribute to producing the disease, I must confess I have not been able to discover anything in the whole morbid process, or any morbid change that cannot be the product of those noxious influences which I consider as the main, if not the exclusive, causes of the disease, and which, in my opinion, are well able to produce every one of those morbid changes, which I had an opportunity to observe. Those injurious influences, or agencies, which I am obliged to consider as the principal causes, act in different ways, for a better survey, may be divided into two classes.

"As belonging to the *first class*, I look upon everything that is apt to cause an interruption of the perspiration, and in the *second class* I place all such noxious influences as are able to interfere, directly, with the process of respiration, and all such foreign substances as enter the respiratory passages, and cause, thereby, congestion and inflammation of the respiratory mucous membranes and of the tissue of the lungs. There are, also, as I have already mentioned, some other minor causes or agencies which contribute, in one case more, in another less, to the development of the disease, or which are able to cause the character of the same to be more typhoid. These I will discuss under the head of aggravating or auxiliary causes, after I shall have disposed of the main or principal causes.

"1. Injurious influences which act as a cause of the disease, by producing an interruption or partial cessation of the perspiration. These influences are numerous, and of much greater importance than one, who looks at them superficially, may be inclined to suppose. The skin of an animal is a very important organ; it not only serves as a protecting tegument, but has also other vital offices which are scarcely of less consequence to the welfare of the animal organism than those of the lungs. The skin discharges, through its pores, a large amount of wasted material, gaseous and fluid, and absorbs aeriform and fluid substances from the outside world. Consequently, it may be looked upon as an organ whose duty it is to supplement the functions of several other organs, but especially those of the lungs and of the kidneys. To ascertain the effect of a total interruption of the functions of the skin upon the animal organism, interesting experiments have been made by Bouley, Magendie, Gerlach, and others. A complete interruption was brought about by covering the skin of various animals with an air-tight coat of varnish, grease, or tar, and the results, according to Gerlach, have been as follows: 'Accelerated pulsation, extraordinary fullness of the arteries until an increased discharge of urine made its appearance, somewhat accelerated breathing, trembling of the whole body, rapid emaciation, great debility, augmented secretion of an albuminous urine of gall (bilifulvin and bitiverdin), and a decrease of the animal temperature. The latter, however, became not very conspicuous before the animal had become emaciated and was near dying. The animals (horses) so treated died in three to ten days.' Pigs coated all over with grease, for the purpose of killing lice, died within a week, and showed the same symptoms.

"2. The office of the skin, at least so far as the processes of elimination and absorption are concerned, bears also a very close relation to the functions of the diverse serous and mucous membranes. It is true, if the skin is disqualified to perform its allotted duties, or if the latter are interrupted by some means, the same will partially be performed, but partially only, by those organs named, the lungs and the kidneys, which, in such a case, will make extraordinary efforts to maintain the equilibrium in the organic change of material, as indispensable to the preservation of health. Still, as I have said, these organs, in addition to their own duties, can only partially perform the functions of the skin; certain parts of the wasted material, constantly produced, will not be discharged, but will remain in the organism. The lungs, the kidneys, the serous and the mucous membranes, if I may use the expression, will be overburdened, and the consequence will be that just those organs will be the first ones that become diseased, or that will have to suffer from over-exertion, and from the injurious effects necessarily produced by a retention of wasted material in the organism, and by a constant loss of organic compounds that cannot be spared. That such a loss is taking place, if the perspiration is interrupted, has been proved by the experiments of Professor Gerlach, which shows that the urine, in such a case, carries off albumen. Further, that such an interruption must necessarily produce a disturbance in the circulation of the blood, which results in an extraordinary flow of blood to those organs—lungs, kidneys, etc.—burdened with increased functions, and constitutes in that way a cause of congestion and subsequent inflammation, is too evident to need any further explanation. At any rate, these facts will be very plain to any one who has ever suffered from any cold.

"Finally, I wish to say a few words in regard to a hygienic mistake committed on almost every farm in the West. I refer to the practice of feeding the swine almost exclusively with corn, a practice which certainly is not calculated to produce healthy and vigorous animals, but which necessarily must result, as I shall try to show, in weakening the organism, and in creating a predisposition to disease. How much or how little this practice has contributed to produce the now-prevailing epizootic influenza of swine, I am not prepared to decide. I have, however, reasons to suppose that this practice has not been without influence. The organism of a domestic animal is composed of about fifteen or twenty elements, or undecomposable constituents of matter, united to numerous organic compounds. A constant change of matter is taking place, and a part of these elements, in the form of organic compounds, is constantly wasted, and carried off by the various processes of secretion and excretion. The organism, therefore, in order to remain healthy, and maintain its normal composition, must receive, from time to time, an adequate supply of those elements, contained in suitable or digestible organic compounds, so as to cover the continual loss, and, if the animal is young, to produce growth and development. The simplest way to introduce the elements into the animal organism is to give food which contains them in nearly the right proportions. A few of these elements besides hydrogen and oxygen, are sometimes in the form of suitable compounds, contained in limited, though very seldom sufficient, quantities in the water for drinking; for instance, calcium (in the form of lime), iron, etc. One important element—oxygen—enters the organism, also, in large quantities through the lungs and through the skin, but all others have to be introduced wholly, or almost wholly, in the form of food. Almost all kinds of fluid, however, milk perhaps excepted, lack some important elements of their composition, contain others in insufficient quantities, and still others in greater abundance than required. Therefore, if such a kind of food is given exclusively—corn, for instance,—which is destitute of some of the mineral elements, and contains only an insufficient quantity of nitrogenous compounds, which are of so great an importance in the animal organization, irregularities and disorders in the exercise of the various functions, and imperfect development of certain parts and organs, will be the unavoidable results.

"One may ask, if the causes of the diseases are of such an ordinary character, how can it be possible that it has become such an extensive epizooty ?—The answer is not very difficult, and an explanation is easily given. At first, notwithstanding the most diligent search and patient inquiry, I have not been able to discover any injurious influences or agencies of a general character besides those enumerated, which, possibly, might have acted as a cause. Secondly, the treatment or the keeping of the swine is essentially everywhere the same in all the Western States. The causes mentioned are, therefore, of a sufficiently universal character to produce an epizootic disease. Our western farmer, as a general rule, careless enough, if possible, in his treatment and care of his horses and cattle, usually thinks a hog is only a "*hog;*" can get along with "*hoggish*" treatment, delights in nastiness, filth, and dirt of any description; does not need a dry, comfortable, and clean resting place during the night, nor clean and fresh water for drinking and bathing; nor shade and shelter against the burning rays of a western sun, against cold dews of the morning, or the sudden changes of weather and temperature in general.

"Somebody may object, and may say, if the principal causes of the disease have their sources in the manner in which the swine are raised and provided for, which does not differ essentially from what has been since the country was first settled, how then does it happen, or how can it be explained, that the disease did make its appearance as an epizooty only a few years ago, and not immediately among the swine of the first settlers, or while the country was yet new, and is now increasing in violence from year to year? This question is not difficult to answer. While the country was new, pig-sties, hog-yards, hog-lots, and pastures, and the places which contained the water for drinking and bathing were not yet contaminated and impregnated to such an extent as they are now with filth and excrement; bare and dusty ground was less abundant, and the number of swine kept together, on one dry place, as a general rule, was a great deal smaller. The disease will increase in malignancy and spread in the same proportion in which dung and dirt is allowed to accumulate, and in which the size of the herds is increased.

"A great many farmers believe, nay, hold themselves convinced, that the epizootic influenza of swine is a contagious disease, and they have kindly furnished me facts which, I admit, point very strongly that way. To tell the truth, I am not yet prepared to decide that question, because such a decision requires numerous experiments, and these I have not been able to make. Still I am inclined to think the epizootic character, or the fearful spreading of the disease, can be explained satisfactorily without the existence of a contagion. The fact that the hogs and pigs running at large in the streets of the cities, with a few exceptions, are healthy, and remain exempted from the disease, goes far to show that the latter is not communicated by a contagion, as animals leading such a vagabond life are, as a general rule, much more exposed to the influence of contagions than any others.

"DURATION OF THE MORBID PROCESS.

"In some cases the disease has had a fatal termination within two days after the first plain symptoms of sickness have made their appearance, and a few cases have been reported to me, in which the animals have died within six or twelve hours; but I am inclined to think the first symptoms have escaped observation—a very common occurrence in diseases of swine. The average duration of the disease may be set down as from five to fifteen days. Still some animals have been sick from three to six weeks, but most of them have recovered, and then a part of that time belongs to the stage of convalescence. Or if the patients have died, the duration of the disease has been protracted by relapses.

"PREVENTION.

"The measures of prevention consist in removing the causes as enumerated above. If this is done, no other special treatment will be required to ward off the disease, and no medicine will be needed. To give medicine to a healthy animal is, under all circumstances, a bad practice, fraught with injury, and should not be done, unless it is intended to destroy injurious influences. To use medicine for the purpose of strengthening the constitution of an animal, is simply folly, as just the opposite will be the result. But to the point: I am confident the epizootic influenza of swine, or the disease improperly called hog cholera, will cease to make its appearance, or, at any rate, will become a very rare occurrence, and will lose its epizootic character, if, first, every large herd of swine is divided into several small herds, or lots, each containing about three or four animals; if, secondly, each lot is provided with a comfortable pen or place to sleep in, which is free from filth, dust, and manure, is well ventilated, and provided with a good roof; if, thirdly, every hog or pig has access, several times a day, or as often as temperature, weather, and circumstances require, to fresh and clean water for drinking and bathing, either in a large trough or in a brook, creek, or streamlet; if, fourthly, no filth, manure, or dirt, is allowed to accumulate in any of the sties, yards, hog-lots, or pastures, in which the hogs or pigs are kept; and if, finally, hogs and pigs receive always a suitable variety of sound healthy food, which is not soiled with dirt or manure. I know very well some farmers will be dissatisfied with my advice, and would have preferred to be sent to the drug store for medicines. Others would think to comply with my prescription will be too much trouble altogether, and some of them may say: 'If we can not keep our hogs any more in the old 'hoggish' fashion, but must treat them like animals ought to be treated, we prefer to keep no hogs at all.' Very well, if they do not keep any hogs, they certainly will not lose any, and their neighbors, who continue to raise swine, and take proper care of them, will be the gainers in a two-fold respect. At first they will reap the benefit from the scarcity of hogs thus produced, and, secondly, they will be amply repaid by their swine for the care bestowed upon them. At any rate, it will pay much better for any one to raise, for instance, fifty hogs, to keep them well in every respect, to lose none, and to develop them to first-class animals, (so-called 'Philadelphia' hogs), than to raise 100 or 200 head, to keep them 'hoggish,' to lose more than fifty to seventy per cent, and to produce animals that figure as 'scalawags' in the market reports. Moreover, the amount of food that is needed to produce 200 pounds of inferior, and frequently unhealthy, pork—if the pig is kept on a manure heap in the barn-yard, or in any nasty hog-lot, and in the old common way and careless fashion—will produce 300 pounds of good healthy, and palatable pork, if the keeping of the animal is always in strict accordance with hygienic laws. If the latter are never violated, the epizootic influenza of swine, I am sure, will not make its appearance; but if the mode of keeping swine is not changed the disease will increase in frequency and in malignancy from year to year.

"TREATMENT.

"The treatment may be divided into two parts—a hygienic and a medical treatment. The former includes a removing of causes, and is alike in many, or even in most, diseases, of the greatest importance. The sick animal must be separated from the herd, and must be provided with a clean, dry, and well ventilated resting place, which is not exposed to drafts of air, and which affords otherwise sufficient protection against heat, cold, and wet. The same, further, must have, besides pure air to breathe, clean water to drink, and healthy and easily digestible food to eat. If the sick animals are thus treated, and the causes promptly removed, a great many sick animals (provided, of course, they are not too far gone) will be saved by proper medical treatment; but if these directions are not complied with, even the best medical treatment will be of very little avail. As to the use of medicines, I would recommend to give to each patient at the beginning of the disease a good emetic, composed either of powdered White Hellebore (*Veratrum album*), or of Tartar Emetic in a dose of about one grain for each month the sick animal is old, if the same is of fair size, but not exceeding sixteen to twenty grains, even if the animal is full-grown or several years old. The emetic is easily administrated by mixing it with a piece of boiled potato, or, if White Hellebore is chosen, (which I consider as preferable), by sprinkling it on the surface of a small quantity of milk. Boiled potato or milk will not be refused by any hog unless the patient is already very sick, or far gone, and in that case it will be too late to give an emetic. After the medicine has taken effect, the animal will appear to be very sick, and will try to hide itself in a dark corner, but in about two or three hours will make its appearance again, and will be willing, in most cases at least, to accept a little choice food, for instance, a boiled potato, a little milk, etc. At that time it will be advisable to give again a small dose of medicine, consisting either of a few grains (two or three, to a full-grown animal, and to a pig in proportion) of Tartar Emetic, or of the same amount of Calomel, also mixed with a piece of boiled potato; or, if appetite should not have returned, mixed with a pinch of flour and a few drops of water, and formed into small round pills. A sick hog, I will remark here, should not be drenched with medicine under any circumstances, for a drench given by force is very apt to pass down the windpipe into the lungs as soon as the animal squeals, and frequently causes instant death. The Tartar Emetic is to be preferred, if the disease has its principal seat in the respiratory organs, or presents itself in its catarrhal rheumatic form; and the Calomel deserves preference if the gastric, or bilious rheumatic form is prevailing, and especially if the liver is seriously affected. Either medicine may be given in such doses as have been mentioned, two or three times a day, for several days in succession, or till a change for the better will be plainly visible. It may also be advisable (but particularly if the typhoid character of the disease is very manifested) to mix for each hog or pig, now and then, a few drops of Carbolic Acid with the water for drinking, or with the slop. Animals that are convalescent, and have been reduced very much by the disease, and are yet weak, should receive, mixed with their food, small doses of Sulphate of Iron, (copperas), say from five to twenty grains, according to age and size, but the use of iron must be discontinued if the patient becomes constipated, or if the excrements turn black. Those convalescents in which the morbid process has produced considerable hepatization of the lungs, will be benefited by giving them repeatedly small doses (from ten to fifty grains) of purified Carbonate of Potash, for the purpose of promoting the absorption of the exudation deposited in the tissue of the lungs.

"Externally, a good counter-irritant, or blister, applied on both sides of the chest, and composed of Cantharides or Spanish flies and Oil (one ounce of the former to four ounces of the latter constitutes the proportion), boiled together over a moderate fire for half an hour, or in a water-bath for half an hour, will produce a very beneficial result, especially in those cases in which the serous membranes of the chest constitute the principal seat of the morbid process. In most cases one application will be sufficient, provided the oil is thoroughly rubbed in and the disease has not made progress too far. If the first application should fail to raise a good blister (swelling and exudation), a second one may be made the next day. In those cases, however, in which the morbid process has made too much headway, or has wrought too much destruction of tissue to admit recovery, the counter-irritant will produce no blister and no swelling whatever, a fact which constitutes a valuable prognostic symptom, for it indicates that the vitality of the animal is already very low, and that a further treatment will be of no avail. Fontanelles or Setons have nearly the same effect as a vesicatory or fly-blister, but act slower, and are less reliable, and may otherwise cause some damage, on account of the typhoid character of the disease, by weakening the constitution of the animal."

In a communication from Dr. Detmers, dated November 30th, 1876, he says:

"Calling every disease of swine 'hog cholera,' has caused a great deal of mischief, and the sooner that name can be abolished the better.

"Anthrax diseases are entirely different from what I found in Missouri," [described in foregoing report].

"There is nothing in common but the epizootic character."

CHAPTER XXV.

SO-CALLED "HOG CHOLERA."

Dr. N. H. Paaren, late State Veterinarian of Illinois, in reference to accounts of fearful ravages of "Hog Cholera" in Missouri and Illinois, writes as follows in regard to this much dreaded scourge :

" * * * The different forms in which anthrax fever develops itself, manifest different symptoms, among which the following are some of the most prevalent : The animals suddenly appear dull, separating themselves from the herd; and totally refusing food and water, they seek dark places, or dig themselves beneath the litter, or into the ground. Symptoms of colic and a disposition to rest on the belly are amongst the signs indicating abdominal pain. Diarrhœa soon sets in ; also occasional violent retching and vomiting. The animal is not able to move freely, on account of weakness in the hind quarters—it staggers, and at last, paralyzed, it cannot move. Deglutition is interfered with, and the breathing is difficult. Painful swellings occur around the throat, extending downwards to the chest, which swelling is hard, hot, and painful. There is also frothing at the mouth and a painful cough, and appearance of boils. Sometime before death a discoloration of the skin appears on the neck, the ears, the back, under the belly, or the inside of the hind extremities, which discoloration, from being at the beginning of a bright-red or purple color, at the last stages of the disease attains a dark-bluish or black color. The visible membranes of the mouth and nose attain a dark livid color, and the mucous membranes of the eyelids and the white front of the eye become dark-red. Death occurs often very suddenly, and in most cases within twelve hours to two or three days. Recovery is seldom, and generally very slow, if ever complete.

"*Post-mortem* examinations reveal, in all cases, the most unmistakable signs of the true nature of this disease. Putrefaction sets in very quickly. The membranes of the nose, mouth, and rectum, are of a dark color. Dark bloody fluid is often observed to ooze from the nose and the rectum. The capillaries and small veins of the skin, as also the tissue under the skin, are of a dark color, and overfilled with dark blood. The bacon, diminished in quantity, is soft, sometimes of a yellowish color, and blood-stained. In animals that die suddenly, the brain and the spinal cord are found overfilled with blood. On opening the abdominal cavity, a most disagreeable and fetid odor escapes; the stomach, the intestines, the liver, and the spleen, are overfilled with blood and yellow serum. The spleen, especially, is large, soft, of a dark color, and overfilled with blood; and the organs of the chest are congested or studded with blood spots. The blood is in a state of dissolution, is of a very dark color, and does not coagulate perfectly.

The causes of the disease are obscure; but as it is more prevalent in low and undrained localities than on high and well-drained soil, it is considered to be due mainly to miasmatic and malarious emanations. Confinement in filthy sties, impure drinking water, and want of change in food, etc., are also amongst the causes. We are convinced that many animals of this class are annually lost from the effects of improper food, or from living in an atmosphere surcharged with poisonous effluvia, the product of animal or vegetable decomposition. Decomposing substances, both animal and vegetable, corn that has undergone a change from long keeping or exposure to damp, and which is loaded, perhaps, with the sporules of poisonous fungi, brine from the meat tub—these and other similar substances are often given to pigs as food, and in many instances have been known to cause very great losses. Much that we have seen convinces us of the necessity of more attention being paid to the quality of the food of these animals than is generally being done, and also to the nature of their lodgings, as well as the air they breathe.

"The treatment is most unsatisfactory, owing to the acute nature of the disease; in fact, all remedies are useless when not administered as soon as the first symptoms appear. When the disease breaks out in a herd, the animals should be kept on low diet, have plenty of exercise and fresh air. In the early stage of the disease cold water sluicings, often repeated, have proved beneficial, and, so has the method of burying in the earth in a cool and dark place. For this purpose a hole is dug, sufficiently large and deep to admit Mr. Pork sidewise, (the legs being previously tied with a soft straw band); the body is then covered with a sufficient quantity of earth and grass turf, leaving the head free; and in order to support the head, a grass turf is laid under the snout. Before burial, several injections, consisting of cold water with vinegar, are thrown into the rectum. In order to keep the surrounding earth constantly cool, cold water is, every half hour, to be let on it. The animal remains thus buried until it recovers, which, in successful cases, happens within six, twelve, or eighteen hours. Hog cholera is treated in many different ways, each having its advocates; some people have seen good effects from bleeding in the earliest stages of this disease. Emetics and purgatives, in connection with lukewarm injections of salt water with vinegar, are very strongly recommended. In the beginning of the disease, success has also attended the administration of an emetic, such as White Hellebore and Ipecacuanha, of each two parts; Tartar Emetic one part; mix and give a small pig a scruple, and a larger one half a drachm, thrown dry upon the root of the tongue; this to be followed up by purgatives and clysters. Purgative to consist of Epsom Salts, one, two or three ounces, according to the size, and age of the animal, administered in broth or swill from a bottle. Exercise, fresh air, and sluicing the animal over with cold water are measures to be recommended. Animals that recover, unless well treated, continue to suffer from partial paralysis, or from rheumatic inflammation of the joints.

"As 'an ounce of prevention is worth more than a pound of cure,' a few remarks concerning this may not be out of place. First of all, avoid, as far as possible, all causes of this malady. Never keep sick and sound animals together; adopt remote separation and close watching. Keep the animals on spare allowance of well-cooked animal food, wholesome diet, fresh and clear water, fresh air and good litter; in fact, cleanliness in every respect is the best preventive against the disease. A few large pieces of rock salt, as well as charcoal, should be kept in the hog pen. Let the hogs have plenty of fresh water, but never run them to and from watering. Don't compel your hogs to drink snow water, if better water is procurable. In hot summer time, keep the hogs under shelter during the hottest hours of the day, especially if hog cholera is prevailing; during which hours, if practicable, and after the hogs are cooled off, give them a good sluicing with cold water, which repeat before letting them out in the afternoon. Unripe fruit and sour milk and water is a good diet in hot weather, but the hogs should not be given more than they can eat at one meal. Besides this, it is advisable, where and when hog cholera exists, to give an occasional emetic. During an existing epidemic, let them vomit every eight days. The best emetic for the hog is White Hellebore, of which give each hog, according to its size, from ten to twenty grains finely powdered. It is best given in the morning, early, before feeding. Mix the doses for each hog in a bucket, with some sour milk, and let him drink it. During that day keep the hogs at home, under shelter, and feed sparingly with some sour milk or unripe fruit. As it is a matter of great importance to keep the bowels in good order, give occasionally some Saltpetre in the drinking water during the following seven days; and—let us repeat it—the hogs must have plenty of fresh and clean water. Prevention by cleanliness and comfort, release from restraint of pens, and the use of salt, tar, coal, ashes, sulphur, etc., have numerous testimonials of efficacy.

"When a destructive disease threatens the animals, and, through them, the most valuable section of our national wealth, it should be the duty of all concerned to obey the dictates of science and experience in order to avert danger and loss. But it must be confessed that to obtain successful results individual efforts go for little. It is on the strict observance of sanitary laws, and to the wise measures prescribed by authority, that reliance must be placed. In the words of an eminent medical writer, 'The day has gone past for an isolated individual or craft to avert pestilence, as Empedocles did when he shut out the sirocco by stopping a mountain-gap, and removed intermittent fevers by changing the course of the river Hypsa.' These large and beneficient operations are in our day reserved for Governments; and our duty is to urge upon Government, by means of our governing bodies, the necessity of undertaking the prevention of epidemic diseases, both among men and animals, to point out the best modes of securing this prevention, and to see that these measures, when become law, are properly carried out. The prevention of epizootic diseases among our domestic animals should be regarded as a political question, involving more or less the well-being of the whole community; not merely affecting those who own or who endeavor to derive profit from rearing animals, but also affecting the public at large, as regards health, the supply of food, and other essentials. In the extension of a disease of this kind, not only is there loss to the individuals who possess the animals, but also to the public, who have not only a diminished quantity or more expensive supply of food, but also often incur the risk of obtaining it of an inferior or injurious quality, or are otherwise inconvenienced.

Almost all the diseases of swine seem to be popularly resolved into 'hog cholera.' Of all diseases of domestic animals, those of this genus are evidently less thoroughly understood than those of any other farm stock. Ideas on the subject are in a singular state of confusion, and remedies are countless in number, and most incongruous in character. If the symptoms were accurately noted, it would probably be found that several kinds of 'hog cholera'

—as every prevalent disease of the hog appears to be called—are uniting in the mischief produced.

Agricultural stock suffers serious neglect. We venture to assert that ninety per cent of the domestic animals of the farm which suffer from disease throughout the United States annually, are never seen by Veterinary Surgeons. It is most singular that the Americans, who have manifested the greatest activity in the promotion of science and the useful arts, have never been able to found a thoroughly efficient Veterinary College. We number among ourselves but few Veterinarians; and most of them—we may say nearly all—have been induced to leave Europe. Is it to be wondered at that our live stock are cut down by disease in a most disastrous manner? Is it to be wondered at that we are now asking how we may remedy an evil which is found to be of far greater importance than we ever before imagined?

Indeed, the ignorance of those who hold foremost positions amongst us on the subject of the amount of disease in the country—the Department of Agriculture, especially—can only be explained by the fact that if we do not search for information regarding mortality amongst stock, we are not in the way of gleaning it at all. Disease is raging frightfully without intermission. Truth must prevail in the end, and no better conformation of what we have said can be obtained than that derived from the state of anxiety and alarm which now exists throughout many portions of our country, where mortality amongst stock is among the daily records of our newspapers the whole year round.

Examples and estimates, after all, give but a slender idea of the devastation, misery, embarrassment and loss that has been, and is due, in very great measure, to the ignorance, apathy and neglect shown by those in authority. We speak but the sentiment of the stock owners and breeders of the country, when we express our earnest regret that the Department of Agriculture pays so little attention to the investigation of the causes and character of the diseases of our domestic animals, in which the interests of all classes of agriculturists are so largely concerned. In view of the great importance of this matter, the great interests at stake, and the prevalence of epidemic diseases among our domestic animals throughout this vast country, it is simply astonishing that the Department of Agriculture contents itself with gathering in the statistics of mortality, utterly neglecting the most important object of recommending or providing remedial means, or institute proper scientific investigations for the benefit of the sufferers and the public at large."

James Law, Professor of Veterinary science in Cornell University, gives the following as the causes, symptoms, and treatment of hog cholera.

"The period of incubation is from seven to fourteen days, but is less in a hot climate.

"*Causes.*—Contagion, privation, starvation, confinement, filth, etc.

"*Symptoms.*—General ill health, shivering, fever, great dullness, prostrating fever, hides under litter, lies on belly, weakness of hind limbs, and later of the fore limbs, rapid, weak pulse, dry snout covered by blood-stained spots, which also cover the skin, eyes, etc., often a hard cough, little or no appetite, intense thirst, tender abdomen. After death, blood-staining infiltrations into lungs and bowels, ulcers on bowels.

Treatment.—Give cooling, acid drinks, Buttermilk, Sulphuric Acid, etc.; feed soft, mucilaginous food, such as Oil-cake. Administer twenty drops of Perchloride of Iron twice a day. Blister the abdomen by means of Mustard and Turpentine; stimulate if very prostrate.

"*Prevention.*—Avoid all debilitating conditions, poor or spoiled food; keep animals constantly thriving. Feed Charcoal or Ashes, also Tar or Carbolic Acid. Avoid contact with disease. Burn infected piggeries and remove to a new place."

In further comments on the disease Prof. Law says:

"Examples, which might be very greatly extended, imply that a sound mixed diet is of great importance in maintaining a healthy activity of the various organic functions, and a vigor to a large extent antagonistic to this and other diseases, and that a somewhat similar immunity may be secured by the use of tonics, antiseptics, and gently stimulating agents. But if we rest our faith upon any or all of these as sure cures or preventives, we shall only pave the way for disappointment whenever the disease takes on an unusually malignant type. Thus, in spite of the protective power of a partially milk diet, as above mentioned, how often does the disease prevail most disastrously in the herds of cheese and butter factories, and, notwithstanding the good effects of an occasional meal of flesh, we find the most extensive losses among pigs that are largely carnivorous, (flesh eating), in their habits.

"Keep your hogs clean is good advice. Protect them from the hot, reeking bed of manure and close sleeping place, where the emanations from decomposing dung, urine, straw and other organic matter are added to those of their own skins and lungs when huddled together in great numbers. See that both food and water are clean, in the sense of being free from disease germs, and from the microscopic particles of decomposing organic matter, which, within the system as well as outside of it, furnish appropriate food for the disease, poison, and favor its increase, while they depress the vital powers and lessen the chances of the virus being thrown off. No less important is the purity of the air, since the delicate membrane of the lungs, perhaps more than any other, furnishes an easy mode of entrance for any injurious external matter. Finally, purity of the blood can only be maintained by a healthy functional activity of all the vital organs, which insures the perfect elaboration of every plastic constituent of the blood, and the excretion of all waste matters that have already served their purpose in the system. By perfect cleanliness, the poison, even if generated or introduced, will be virtually starved out as surely as an army in a closely besieged fortress. But it will be observed that this implies the separation of sound from diseased animals, and the free use of disinfectants, (solutions of sulphate of iron and chloride of lime, fumes of burning sulphur, etc.), to purify the air and other surrounding objects, as well as the simple clearing away of filth. And it is here that the pork-raisers are most frequently at fault. Fifty or a hundred pigs are allowed to crowd together in a filthy manure heap, a rotten straw stack, or under a barn subjected to the droppings of other animals, as well as their own products. Their feeding troughs and drinking water are so supplied that they can get into them with their filthy feet, and they must devour the most obnoxious matter or starve. If, under this abuse, disease is developed, the healthy are left with the sick, as 'they will all have it any way,' and the result is usually a clean sweep. When hog cholera exists, the sick should be placed by themselves under a special attendant, and under the free use of disinfectants ; the healthy should be carefully watched, and on the first sign of illness, as increased temperature, to be ascertained by the introduction of a clinical thermometer into the rectum, they should be at once taken from the herd and carefully secluded. This, with active disinfection, will enable the owner to cut short an outbreak. and save perhaps the great majority of an already infected herd, Again, the sale of animals from an infected stock, to be removed from the premises alive, should be severely punished, and the disinfection of the buildings where the sick have been, should be made imperative. We shall obtain the greatest success with this disease when we treat it as a contagious malady, and whenever it is found to exist, give our main attention to prevent the further generation and dissemination of the poison."

The following is collated from the correspondence of the *Prairie Farmer*, and coming direct from men emphatically practical, it is well worthy consideration. Mr. John S. Bowles, of Hamilton, Ohio, writing to that journal in November, 1872, for information about Hog Cholera, says:

"I will now describe the disease of which my hogs are dying, and of which a great portion of the hogs in this vicinity are also dying.

"The first symptom is a dullness or sleepiness in the actions of the hog. He walks to his food instead of running. He holds his head down within two or three inches of the ground, and should he raise it, he holds it slightly to one side. He eats his food as though he had no appetite for it. He does not lie down with his fellow hogs, but mopes about, lying by himself, often in the sun instead of the shade. After the disease progresses a little, the hog refuses to eat altogether. His ears swell. Sometimes a little purple-colored blood will run from his nose. Sometimes, but not in the majority of cases, he will have a diarrhœa. If he is a white hog, his ears and the lower part of his throat and between his fore legs turn to a purple hue. Sometimes he dies in two days, and sometimes he lingers for two weeks. The latter part of his illness he heaves at his flanks, having what is called the 'Thumps.' He is also very weak in his hind quarters. When he is driven up he starts with a squeal, as though much frightened, and runs off reeling on his hind legs, with his nose nearly down to the ground.

"This season is the first one I have ever been troubled with hog cholera, and I have every reason to believe the disease originated on my own farm.

"There were diseased hogs all through the neighborhood for two months previous to mine taking the disease, but I do not think mine had any contact with any of them, or in fact with any hogs but their fellows.

"The disease broke out in my hogs in a field which has a stream of spring water running through it. It is an old sugar camp, nine-tenths cleared, but the hogs could be in the shade all the time if they wished.

"The rest of the field, where there were no sugar trees, is a clover pasture. There was no filthy beds, or pens, or bad water in the case—on the contrary, quite the reverse.

"At the same time I had 44 hogs taken from the same lot as these store hogs, that were in three board pens, side by side. These hogs were being fed all the old corn they would eat, and had been up about three weeks when the others took the cholera. Although they lay considerably in their own filth, and had a large manure heap on one side of them, none of them took the cholera; for four weeks it broke out among their adjoining fellows, and until 18 of them had died. Now one (only), of the fattening hogs is sick.

"The hogs in which the disease broke out had been on clover pasture, alone, during the early part of the summer. As I had more hogs than clover, I soon fed them three ears of corn per day, each. After harvest, I turned the hogs on the wheat and barley stubble, and quit feeding them corn. When the stubble gave out, I commenced feeding the hogs three stalks of grain corn per day each, corn being just out of the milk.

"There was then abundance of clover pasture as all my stubbles were sown with clover. I wanted, however, to keep my hogs in the same condition they were until my new crop of corn was sufficiently ripened to feed them for fattening.

"In about two weeks they commenced dying, and out of about 99, averaging 160 to 170 pounds, I have lost 19, and several more are sick. Thinking the green corn had something to do with the disease, I sold 41 of the healthiest to a neighboring distillery, and went to feeding the remainder with dry old corn. They seem to do better since I changed their diet—that is, they do not die so fast.

"I have an idea that green corn, second growth clover, etc., have a tendency to *excite* the disease, though I think the primary cause is something similar to malaria.

"Can you give me any information on the subject?

"N. B.—Besides the 19 hogs, averaging 160 lbs., I have lost about 20 spring pigs, and 30 odd sucking pigs."

In a later issue, "A. M. W.," of Odin, Illinois, says:

"In your issue of last Saturday is a communication asking the experience and advice of other farmers as to hog cholera. I have been keeping hogs ever since the disease first began to be heard of in the West, have been cleaned out several times by it, and therefore gladly communicate something of what I know about it. The symptoms he describes are exactly the same that I understand to indicate hog cholera. My hogs have taken it when they had free access to the woods and hazle-brush, and all (with the exception of a few old brood sows) have gradually died off. Then again they have had the disease when confined to the fields, not clover, but stubble and timothy meadows, and it has generally commenced its attack soon after harvest, and was the most fatal about the time the most green corn was fed, though I don't think the corn had anything to do with it.

"Now for the remedies. I have been clear of it for several years, and for two years before that time, I stopped its ravages at once by administering a prescription that was published in your paper After stopping the disease with that medicine the second time, I saw again in *The Farmer* a prescription recommended as a preventive, and have used that since according to directions, and have had no symptoms of hog cholera in my herd. I don't affirm that either is a specific, but such, as related, were the results; hence, of course, I have great faith in the medicine, and have no fears of cholera now in raising hogs. There may be others of your readers who have had experience with those medicines. If they have failed or otherwise, they would certainly do their brother farmers a favor by communicating the fact. I have the recipe for the cure in my scrap book, cut from *The Prairie Farmer* at the time, to date. It is: Sulphur, 2 lbs.; Copperas, 2 lbs.; Madder, 2 lbs.; Black Antimony, ½ lb.; Saltpetre, ½ lb.; Arsenic, 2 oz. The quantity is sufficient for 100 hogs, and is mixed with slop enough for a few doses all round—a pint to each hog. Each time I tried this, I had about 50 head, and not one died that was able to walk to the trough and had enough life left to drink.

"The preventive was published by Prof. J. B. Turner, in 1862, in *The Prairie Farmer*, and then again two years or more ago he sent you the same recipe with some characteristic remarks, affirming his continued reliance on its efficacy, which you published at the time. The paper was mislaid, and I wrote to Mr. T., and here is his

Recipe.—One peck of Wood-ashes, four pounds Salt, one pound Black Antimony, one pound Copperas, one pound Sulphur, quarter-pound Saltpetre. Pound and mix thoroughly; moisten enough to prevent waste; put in a trough in a dry place where the hogs can at all times eat just as much as they please of it. If predisposed to cholera, they will eat it very freely, and it will make something of an item of expense, for a time; at other times they will eat less, or perhaps none at all."

Some time after the appearance of the above letter, Mr. John G. Dutrich, of Normal, Illinois, wrote:

"In *The Farmer* of December 14, 1872, there was an article on hog cholera, written and sent to you by A. M. W., of Odin, Ill. It came to me just in time to save my lot of one hundred shotes and hogs, and a nicer lot of the former could not have been found in the country a week before the article reached me. But that week took out about fifteen of the choice ones. I will only say that I used the remedy as soon as I could get it, and have only lost one by cholera since, and that one would not drink."

Respecting the preventive, the venerable Prof. Turner himself, says:

"I know of no one who has had any hog cholera of account from that day, (1862), who has persistently made use of it in advance of the appearance of disease. I have heard of hogs being actually cured, after disease sets in, by being scrubbed all over daily with Copperas water moderately strong.

"Hogs should at all times be supplied with stone coal, as they will then eat less of the above mixture, and be less expense."

Mr. A. C. Moore, the eminent Illinois breeder of Poland-Chinas, says, in his *Swine Journal:*

"Of this disease, which has proved so fatal, at different times within the last twelve years, in nearly every locality, especially in the Mississippi Valley, much has been said, and much written. Many believe the inciting causes are to be found in the want of some mineral elements in the soil of this great, once-submerged valley; but there are many theories as to its causes, and all of them are more or less substantiated by facts. It seems to present itself at different times and places, under varying symptoms. The first indications differ.

"Though I have never had a case of this scourge among my hogs, I have carefully examined the first appearances on several occasions when it has visited neighboring yards and farms. The first symptoms that I have seen, in cases considered to be cholera, were these: the eyes looked hollow, and deep set in the head; the hair seemed to raise, or rough up; there was a gathering of a dark-looking substance in the inner corner of the eye; these were followed by the skin looking rough and scaly, and of a dark-red color; then came vomiting and diarrhœa, more or less frequent, according to the violence of the attack. In many cases, there is a short and very difficult breathing, the head drops or is held to one side, and a cough shows itself; the cough being peculiar in this—that the animal *stops* to cough, and puts his nose quite near to the ground, in fact, it seems as though he could not cough while walking, as is usually done with a common cough. The hog seems indisposed to move, is stiff and 'drawn up.' There are other morbid conditions which are ascribed to cholera, but the truth seems to be that these conditions vary so much, and the indications or first symptoms are so different, that I am compelled to believe that there are many ailments called cholera that are not cholera. It is therefore that so many quack nostrums can get certificates of cure from farmers, whose stock has perhaps been cured, but cured from what? They believe it cholera, and so certify, but when the same remedy is given to a herd that actually have that disease, then it fails; such failure is not usually reported beyond the immediate neighborhood.

"I know it does not matter to the loser what the disease may be called that takes away his herd, so far as his loss is concerned, but until the observing and scientific world have more agreement as to the causes and conditions of this dread disease, it may be in vain that we proclaim any remedy to be a specific cure. In case of actual attack from this disease, (having no experience,) I should at once conclude that, so far as the diseased animal was concerned, the preventives and conditions hereinafter named, had not reached the individual case, either from my neglect to provide them at all, or in sufficient quantities, and I would apply them at once, with thoroughness. I would also give an ounce of *Carbolic Acid*, well dissolved, and mixed in slop for every twenty-five head of my herd, and repeat this dose every two or three days, carefully noting conditions and changes. Above all things, remove an affected hog at the first positive symptoms, to a yard or pen, if not by himself, at least entirely separated from the well hogs. Dispose of every carcass at once, and remove all filth of an infectious nature. If it be true, as claimed by some, that there is no *specific remedy* for this disease, it certainly follows that the 'ounce of prevention' must be thoroughly applied.

"For all general purposes of health, and as a preventive from disease, I have, for many years, used the following mixture with uniform and marked benefit. Take 1 bushel Charcoal, small pieces; 3 bushels Wood-ashes; ½ bushel slacked Lime; ½ bushel Salt; 2 lbs. Spanish brown; 5 lbs. Sulphur; ½ lb. Saltpetre; ½ lb. Copperas. Pulverize the last two thoroughly; mix all in a bin, box, or barrel, and keep in an open trough, where the hogs can have free access to it, and keep well moistened with good swill, or milk. If your herd is not large, or you lack a sufficient amount of some of the ingredients, mix smaller amounts of each in the same proportion. Aim to keep these articles on hand at all times, and do not neglect their use;

they contain certain chemical elements which are wanting in every hog predisposed to disease. You will soon observe, by careful watching, that the animal that looks the worst, and with which, as you say, 'there seems to be something the matter,' these are the ones that will call on you to fill this trough the oftenest, and they will usually visit it, either as they go to or return from their feed.

"A disease called the cholera sometimes manifests itself by a short and quick, difficult breathing; the head droops, the back is raised, no disposition to move, eyes look bad, a slight cough, of course no appetite; often diarrhœa attends the last stage, in which many animals die. In such symptoms, I would try the *Oil of Peppermint*, prepared as *an essence, but one-third stronger*. Put this into warm water, sweetened with sugar, and give two tablespoonfuls to each of your hogs sick, or subject to attack. A customer, in whose word and observation I have perfect confidence, writes me that he used this remedy in nineteen cases that were affected as above, and not one died, though every hog was lost on the adjoining farm that was attacked, though many other remedies were used."

A correspondent of the Louisville *Courier-Journal* furnishes the following as an "infallible remedy" for Hog Cholera:

"Dissolve thoroughly one pound of Copperas in three gallons of warm water, and apply the wash about milk-warm to the affected animal, by dipping into the solution or rubbing upon it until the skin is thoroughly wet. Whenever the skin of the hog begins to look rough and scaly, or of a dark-red color, apply the wash immediately. Do not wait until the more alarming symptems (vomiting and purging) set in. Apply the wash every day, until the scales are removed."

Seeing accounts in the agricultural press, of the success of the Messrs. R. Kimberly & Son, breeders of Chester Whites, at Green River, Henry county, Illinois, in preventing diseases in their swine, by a simple—and, as they believe, infallible—remedy, we applied to them for particulars.

Under date of March 1st, 1877, they write:

"We have reports from every quarter, of cholera among swine, to an extent that is truly alarming. When we go to a market town, we see load after load of hogs that have died of cholera, and we know that it is raging on every hand, while at the same time, our own herd continues healthy.

"Common 'Smart-weed' tea has prevented, and we believe will prevent—if used judiciously and in season—not only cholera, but the many diseases known by that name.

"In its green state, we pound the Smart weed in an iron kettle, press out the juice and mix it, in small quantities, with good swill.

"When we discover want of appetite in a hog (that is the first symptom in nearly all diseases of swine), we feed them enough of this to make them cough and sneeze greatly, and it has never failed, with us, to bring them around all right.

"We most fully believe that this remedy will not only prevent all cholera, but promote health and thrift.

"For use through the year the herb should be gathered when in bloom, tied in small bundles, and hung in a sheltered, dry place, and when wanted for use, make a tea of it, by boiling. There are two kinds of Smart-weed, and the smallest, with the narrowest leaves, is the one we use.

"We would not part with this remedy for any that has yet been discovered, or is likely to be, for the next twenty years, especially as a preventive and general corrective.

"Disease, however, will continue to carry off a portion of the hogs in the country, so long as they are permitted to pile together in large numbers, in manure heaps, under some old barn or shed, until in a more than fever heat, out of which they rush into a zero atmosphere at feeding time."

Milton Briggs, author of *The Western Farmer and Stock Grower*, and widely known as a successful grower of cattle and hogs on a large scale in Iowa, writes:

"I supply all my hogs with a compound of Bituminous Coal, Wood-ashes, or Lime and Salt. I place in a bin or box, open, so that hogs can dig out at bottom, and not run on to their feed. I place this bin so they can have access to it at all times. Five tons of what is called Slack Coal, with four or five bushels of Lime, or three to four barrels of Wood-ashes and one barrel of Salt, all mixed. This quantity will feed 100 head of hogs about four months. All hogs having access to this feed, will keep free from disease, even if exposed to hogs having the cholera. I have purchased hogs that were diseased, having cholera in its first stages, and turned in with well hogs where there were large numbers running together. All symptoms of disease would soon disappear under this mode of treatment. The cholera hogs would soon begin to cast off their mange or scales from the skin, and assume a healthy appearance. A composition of Carbonate of Soda, Sulphur, Sulphate of Iron, and Carbolic Acid, will arrest the spread of cholera, in its worst stages."

Ezra Stetson, of Neponset, Illinois, a practitioner of medicine for twenty years, and for the twenty years prior to 1876, a farmer and hog raiser on a large scale, by request of the editor presented his views and extended observations on the so-called Hog Cholera in a series of papers carefully prepared for the *National Live Stock Journal*, and he is confident the disease is of the same nature and origin as typhus fever in man, and belongs to a class of diseases caused by what he terms "crowd poison."

He has never known nor heard of an outbreak of this disease, except where large numbers of swine were kept together, unless communicated by contagion.

"It is only when the herd reaches into hundreds that the disease assumes its most malignant form and carries death and destruction in its path like a whirlwind." Extreme heat and cold are favorable periods for it; but it is prevalent all the year, and few animals escape that are exposed to its contagion. Dogs, wolves, and all rapacious animals or birds spread it, and to effectually prevent this, the dead hogs should be wholly consumed by burning.

Dr. Stetson thinks prevention is the only hope, and this must be accomplished by giving hogs proper accommodations, preventing their piling together, insuring them ventilation, shelter from sun, and protection from cold. "Medicines, as such, should never be given them. No specific for this sty fever in swine, or typhus in man, has yet been discovered.

"Disinfectants are the nearest approach to safety from crowd poison that we yet possess. The most valuable is Carbolic Acid, and since using this—eight or ten years—in my own herd, I have suffered no loss from this disease. The crude acid, a dark, tarry liquid, costing about one dollar per gallon, is used at the rate of a pint to a bucket of water, and with this the nests and woodwork about them are sprinkled at least once a week. An ounce of the acid is occasionally put in a barrel of swill or water for the hogs to drink."

At a meeting of stock-breeders and farmers of Iowa, held at West Liberty, during three days in February, 1877, there was an extended discussion on swine management. Mr. J. S. Long, of Jasper county, referring to hog cholera, said he could give some experience that he thought would be of value to all. Years ago he lost thousands of dollars' worth of hogs, but for the last six years he had not lost any, and he had a remedy, if any one would try, he would warrant they would lose no more hogs, provided they did exactly as he said, and the hogs were not past drinking, so they could not take the medicine. He had tried it in thousands of cases, and never had a failure; was now engaged in buying lots of hogs where cholera prevailed; bought 250 recently, and found no trouble in curing them. His remedy was this: "Make Concentrated Lye into good soap by the usual rule; take one pail of the Soap to fifty hogs; put it in a kettle, add water and two pounds of Copperas, boil it, then add dish-water and milk (or anything to make it taste good) till you have about what the fifty hogs will drink. Place enough of the mixture, while warm, for twenty-five hogs to drink, in troughs, in a separate lot. Just as you are ready to let the hogs in, scatter two pounds of Soda in the troughs, the object is to have it foaming as the hogs come to drink. Be sure that every hog drinks, and if he will not drink, put him in the hospital, and if you cannot get him to drink then, knock him in the head, for he will give the cholera to the rest. After twenty-five have had all they will, drink let in twenty-five more, and continue till the whole are treated. The next day I go through with the same operation. After the second day skip a day, then give for two days, and you may turn them out cured. I generally give the same dose once a week to my hogs. An important point is to make the hog drink, and, if he will not take it any other way, add new milk, or put in sugar."

As evidence of his entire faith in his remedy and mode of administering it, Mr. Long offered "to pay ten cents a pound for every hog he could not cure, provided the hog was not past drinking."

CHAPTER XXVI.

VARIOUS DISEASES COMMON TO SWINE.

While in the great pork-producing States the disease, or diseases, known as "Hog Cholera," overshadows in importance all other ailments of swine, there are numerous other diseases to which these animals are more or less subject. Some of these, such as Trichina and Measles, are of greater importance, from their effects upon man than for their injury to the swine themselves, and on this account call for vigilance in preventing them—as cure is out of the question. The leading diseases are here enumerated, and those remedies that have been found most useful are prescribed.

WORMS.

There is perhaps no animated existence that is troubled to so great an extent, or with so many varieties of worms, as the hog. Although savoring, somewhat, of quackery in principle, it is yet almost safe to say that, when your hog is sick, and you cannot tell what is the matter, *doctor for worms.*

"The principal symptom is a gormandizing appetite, without corresponding improvement in flesh, with an excessive itching, causing the animal to rub, especially the hind parts.

"One, known as the round worm, is usually the size of a small goose-quill, and six or seven inches in length, of a brownish color, and somewhat corrugated.

"Probably the most effectual remedy that can be used is Santonin. This is the active principle of a plant called Worm-seed, and is the base of many of the vermifuges. It is in small white crystals, is usually very prompt in its action, and may be given in doses of one-third of a teaspoonful morning and evening, for two or three days, and following with a brisk cathartic, such as Calomel, in teaspoonful doses.

"Two other worms inhabit the lower bowels, or large intestines, generally near the anus, and may be frequently seen coming from the animal. One is a white slender worm, about three inches long, and as large as a knitting-needle; the other a little white worm, shaped somewhat like a tadpole, and half or three-quarters of an inch long.

"Occasionally, these may be removed by giving one and a half tablespoonfuls of Barbadoes Aloes, with one teaspoonful of Copperas, each morning, for a week.

"If this fails to discharge them, after taking three or four days, an injection may be given, as follows: Tincture of Assafœtida, one tablespoonful; Salt, one teaspoonful; Water, half a pint; mix all together, warm silghtly, and inject.

"Such treatment as this may not be appreciated by the reader. But in these days, when a choice breeding animal may cost two or three hundred dollars, we certainly should know all the remedies that may be required to save life or restore health."—(*Dr Chase.*)

Mr. Moore says:

"To swine that are troubled with worms, mix Wood-ashes with Soap-suds, and feed once a week with their slops."

TRICHINA SPIRALIS.

This is a minute worm scarcely visible to the naked eye, that infests the flesh and muscles of man, the hog, and several other animals, such as dogs, cats, rats, and mice, and it was estimated by Leuckart that a single ounce of cat flesh, observed by him, must have harbored more than 300,000 of these parasites, which shows that under favorable conditions they accumulate in immense numbers.

They vary in length from $^1/_{18}$ to $^1/_8$ of an inch, have a rounded slender body, with the head very narrow and sharply pointed, and although so diminutive, are among the most deadly worms known.

The mature and fertile worm lives in the intestines of animals, the immature in minute cysts (sacks or pouches) in the muscles, (see fig. 12), and these cysts only reach maturity and reproduce their kind when the animal they infest is devoured by another, and they are set free by the processes of digestion. Swine permitted to eat the offal from slaughter-houses, carrion, rats, mice, and decaying animal matter of any kind, are usually more or less infested with trichina, and its dangerous nature is a powerful argument in favor of supplying them with food that is sound and wholesome.

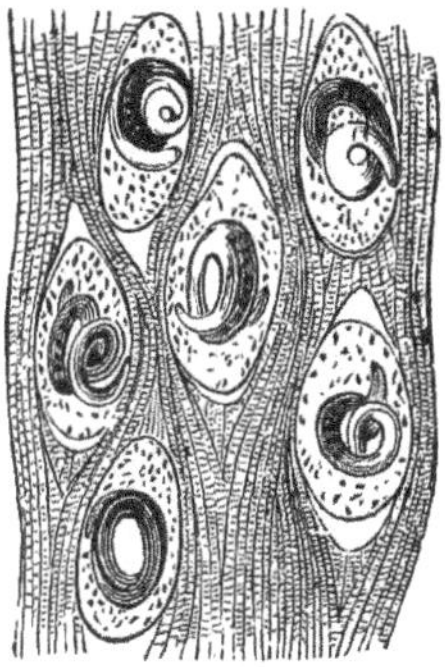

Fig. 12. — TRICHINA IN MUSCLE.—*Magnified.*

In about two days from the time the trichina is taken into the stomach, it reaches the adult condition, and about the seventh day the female brings forth a numerous brood of minute hair-like larvæ which soon begin piercing the intestinal walls, whence they proceed through the system, until they reach and penetrate the muscles. Their borings cause violent muscular pains, like rheumatism, for which in man it is often mistaken; also stiffness, some fever, with diarrhœa, and much irritation for the first fortnight. The duration of an attack is from four to eight weeks, and the period of recovery as much longer. If the patient survives six weeks, recovery may be looked for, as irritation ceases when the worms have become encysted in the muscle.

An attack of trichiniasis where not at first suspected, is liable to be mistaken for typhoid fever.

We have no knowledge of an instance where swine have been lost by being infested with trichina, and the treatment of human subjects so affected has been by the most skilled physicians considered far from satisfactory. Those most familiar with the symptoms recommend, especially at first, cathartics and vermifuges ; Castor Oil, Glycerine, Benzine, Alcohol, and Picric Acid are named.

Hogs that run at large, or are treated with neglect, are always liable to have trichina, and the flesh of such can only be eaten with safety after it is *thoroughly cooked,* and we have seen it authoritatively stated that these disgusting parasites will survive 140 degrees Fahrenheit.

Partially cooked ham, sausage, and similar meats, such as are kept on sale at cheap restaurants, eating stalls, booths, etc., should especially be avoided.

KIDNEY WORMS.

Symptoms: Imperfect use of hind legs, inclination to lie down, a seeming paralysis of hind parts, inability to raise on the hind feet.

Dr. Chase, in his work, "The Hog, its Diseases, and Treatment," says :

"This worm infests hogs to an alarming extent, and though not fatal in its effects, is a frequent cause of disease.

"When full-grown, it is as large as a small wheat-straw, and nearly two inches in length. It inhabits the leaf-lard, in the neighborhood of the kidneys, and we have sometimes seen scores of them in the same hog. It is nearly black along the back, and of a brown color on the belly. It burrows along through the fat, and is a frequent cause of weak loins, and sometimes produces a slight inflammation of the kidneys. Turpentine is the only remedy we have ever found to be of benefit, and conclude that its rapid absorption into the circulation and through the kidneys, has the effect of driving the worm further away from those organs, when the irritation ceases. There is no way of expelling the worm from the system that we are aware of."

Dr. Paaren says in the *Prairie Farmer:*

"Kidney worm is not a common disease in hogs. Occasionally one or two in a number of hogs may suffer from the presence of one or more worms in the kidneys; but the ailment is not often fatal, and becomes so only after a longer time of suffering, and consequent disease or degeneration of one or both kidneys. When we are told that a number of pigs simultaneously refuse their food, lie down, become partly paralyzed, or suffer from spasmodic twitchings, we are inclined to conclude that they are affected with some other ailment than kidney worms."

An old farmer, of La Salle county, Illinois, writes:

"I lately saw inquiries about kidney worms in hogs, indicated by the loss of the use of the hind legs, etc. This disease has prevailed very extensively here, but we now have a certain cure, viz: One tablespoonful of Turpentine poured on across the loins or small of the back, every day, for three days. I have never known it to fail, even when the hogs had been down for weeks unable to rise."

"H. D. Court, the well-known breeder of Chester White swine at Battle Creek, Mich., writes that he has found a teaspoonful of pulverized Copperas, mixed with an equal quantity of Sulphur, fed in the night's meal, for three days, effective in this disease. Sometimes a longer treatment is necessary."

Corn soaked in lye made from wood-ashes, is a convenient preventive, and is used with success when signs of the complaint first appear. Prof. Law says its presence in the kidney may sometimes be recognized by the existence of microscopic eggs in the urine. The same results from another worm—*Eustrongylus gigas.* But without observation of such eggs, weakness of the hind parts cannot be ascribed to *kidney worm.*

MEASLES.

Prof. Law, in his "Farmer's Veterinary Adviser," says:

"The bladder-worm of pork (*Cysticercus cellulosæ*) is the immature form of a tape-worm in man, (*Tænia solium*), and is only caused by pigs having access to human excrement, or to places near privies, etc., from which the segments of the human tape-worm may travel. The cysts, respectively about the size of a grain of barley, are found in the muscles, in the loose connective tissue, and under the skin, in

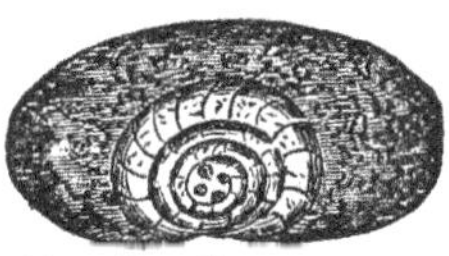

Fig. 13.—CYSTICERCUS CELLULOSÆ.

the serous membranes, in the eye, under the tongue, etc., of swine. [Fig. 13 shows a separate cyst, enlarged; fig. 14, gives the cysts of the natural size as they appear in measly pork.]

"They are also found in this undeveloped form in the muscles, brain, etc., of man, causing disease and death. To man, the para-

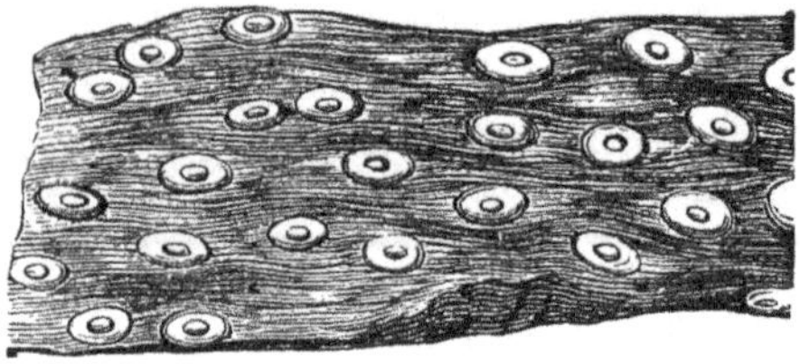

Fig. 14.—CYSTS OF MEASLES IN PORK.

site is usually conveyed by eating under-done pork, or in the cystic form he receives it as the egg in his food (salads, etc.,) and water.

"SYMPTOMS.—In pigs, the cysts can usually be seen under the tongue, or in the eye. In man, there are the general symptoms of intestinal worms, and the passage of the ripe segments.

"Other symptoms may attend the presence of the cysts, accord-

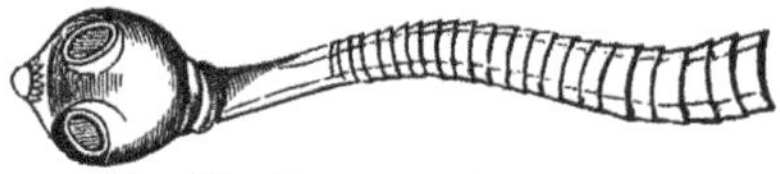

Fig. 15.—HEAD OF TÆNIA SOLIUM.

ing to the organ which they invade. Thus, when passing into the muscles, there are pains and stiffness, resembling rheumatism; when into the brain, coma, stupor, imbecility, delirium, but when they have once become encysted, they may continue thus indefinitely, without further injury.

"TREATMENT.—The cysts scattered through the body are beyond the reach of medicine.

"PREVENTION.—Human beings harboring tape-worms should be compelled to take the measures to expel them. Their stools should be burned, or treated with strong mineral acids. Swine should be kept far apart from all human excrement; no such manure should be used as a top-dressing on pastures open to swine, or on lands devoted to the raising of vegetables to be eaten raw.

"Avoid raw meat, especially pork, even if salted and smoked, and under-done meat and sausages, also well-water, from gravelly soils, in the vicinity of habitations."

MANGE.

"Mange, itch, or scab, in the lower animals is a skin disease of a purely local nature, due to an insect, which induces irritation, ulceration, suppuration, and incrustation on the surface of the body generally. It is a contagious disease, never originating spontaneously, and requiring for its development the passage of the parasites or their eggs from diseased to healthy animals. In man, this disease is termed 'the itch,' and in the lower animals it is usually alluded to as 'mange,' and in sheep it is well known as a fearfully destructive disease, under the name of 'scab.'

"There are some important points in the history of scabies which apply to this disease, as it affects the animal kingdom generally. There is no species in the class *mammalia* that is not attacked with an insect inducing such a disease, if we perhaps except those that live mostly in water. It has been ascertained that though the weak, dirty, and ill nourished condition of some animals renders them very liable to the disease, they only become affected when diseased animals accidentally come in contact with them. A most important point, very clearly established, is, that although any animal may accidentally be the carrier of a contagion between other two, such as a cat or a dog carrying disease from one horse to another, that it is essential for the development of a real scabies on any animal, that the insect should be proper to that animal. Thus human beings, engaged around mangy horses, carry the malady from one animal to another, and suffer but very slightly, and only for a very short time, themselves. The parasite which lives on the horse does not live on man, and the parasite that lives on the sheep does not contaminate the shepherd's dog, though the latter may, like the shepherd, or the many rubbing-places on driftways, be the means whereby the malady spreads.

"The mange of the pig is due to the presence of a burrowing sarcoptes. *Sarcoptes suis* is much like the human sarcoptes and the horse sarcoptes. Itch and mange are known to be essentially skin diseases, curable alone by topical remedies; and the medicines used are valuable almost in proportion to the rapidity with which they destroy the life of the parasites which give rise to the irritation and other morbid appearances.

"In treating the mange, we should first cover the body with soft soap, and wash it off some time afterwards with warm water, and have the animal well brushed; or a wash may be used, consisting of one part of Caustic Potash to fifty parts of water; or one part of Creosote to forty parts of oil, well mixed; or Sulphuret of

Potassium in water, in the proportion of one to ten parts; or a decoction of Tobacco, in the ratio of one to twenty-five; or lastly, concentrated Vinegar. One or two days after the thorough application of either one of these preparations, wash the body well with soap and water or potash lye. Whenever scabies is treated, it is essential to purify all objects with which animals can come in contact. Thus, all rubbing-places and sties should have a covering of lime, or chloride of lime. The sties should be cleaned out entirely, or the pigs removed for a few months to a new pen." (*Dr. Paaren, V. S.*)

RECIPE FOR MANGE OINTMENT.—Melt half a pound of common Turpentine with a pound and a half of Lard. Stir well therein a pound of Flowers of Sulphur, and when cool, rub down upon a marble slab, two ounces of strong Mercurial Ointment with these.

LICE.

"Lice are a sad torment to poverty-stricken and badly-kept stock, appearing by myriads, and causing excessive itching and irritation. They will effectually prevent an animal from laying on fat or doing well, as long as their presence is permitted. Various remedies and dressings are recommended for lice, and some are excessively dangerous, especially the preparations of mercury and arsenic,—the skin of most animals being extremely sensitive to the action of these agents. We have frequently recommended the following formula, as being both safe and destructive to lice: Stavesacre seed, four ounces; White Hellebore, one ounce; boiled in a gallon of water until only two quarts remain. Apply with a brush to the parts where lice are seen. A decoction of Tobacco may also be tried. On no account should mercurial or arsenical preparations be employed in these cases, as, from the great extent of surface it is often necessary to apply the dressing to, death has frequently resulted."—(*Paaren.*)

"We have used the following remedy, which will clean off the lice in two days: Put about one gill of kerosene oil in any old dish, and with a paint brush or old woolen rag rub the oil up and down the back of the animal, and behind the fore leg, and on the flank. Be particular about the last two places, for it is where the lice deposit their eggs, which, if not destroyed, will hatch out in about five days. If it be a black hog, these eggs can be plainly seen, being about the size of timothy seed, and laying close to the skin fast to the hair. No one need fear to use the oil freely, as it will not injure the hog in the least."

"A Tennessee Agricultural paper says: 'W. S. Swann informs us that he has an infallible remedy for ridding hogs of lice, simple and easy of application; which is to take buttermilk and pour it along the hog's back and neck, and after two or three applications, not a louse will be seen. He has tried, and seen it tried, in several cases, with the same success in every instance. Mr. Swann being a reliable man, and the remedy very simple, we recommend its trial to our farmer friends whose hogs are troubled with lice.'"

"A. C. Moore says: 'Take two parts of Kerosene and one part of Lard-oil, mix, and apply to the hair and skin with a sponge or cloth; rub it well over all the parts where nits are liable to be found, and you have a certain cure. Two or three applications, if thoroughly done, will not fail. Be careful to cover the skin behind the ears and fore arms—here are the nits, and these are the places to attack.'"

"B. T. S., Mount Pleasant, Iowa, writes: 'Scotch snuff and hog's lard will destroy lice on hogs. One-fourth pound of Snuff and one and a fourth pound of Lard is sufficient for twenty head. Rub the mixture along the back of the hog with the hand.'"

PNEUMONIA.

This disease is sometimes spoken of as "Thumps," but is more severe and rapidly fatal. Designating it as Inflammation of the Lungs gives a better idea of its seat and nature.

Its symptoms are loss of appetite, shivering, labored breathing, and severe cough. For treatment give the animals warm, comfortable quarters, free access to fresh, cool water, and every morning two drachms Saltpetre, or half an ounce of Hyposulphite of Soda in a small mess of gruel.

In this, as other diseases, feeding much dry corn is detrimental to recovery.

COMMON COUGH.

This is known to many farmers as *rising of the lights.* It is sometimes quite troublesome, if not fatal. The prominent indications of the disease are loss of appetite, incessant and distressing cough, and heaving at the flanks.

As soon as the first symptoms are perceived, the animal should be bled; the palate is the best place; purgatives must then be given, but cautiously. Epsom Salts and Sulphur will be best, administered in a dose of from two to four drachms each, according to the size of the animal; afterwards give a sedative, composed of Digitalis two grains, Pulvis Antimonialis six grains, Nitre half drachm. Cleanliness, warmth, and wholesome, cooling, nutritious food, are likewise valuable aids in combating this disease.

E. W. Bryant, of Illinois, breeder of Poland-Chinas, says, "my remedy for cough in pigs is oats. Feed once or twice a week all they will eat. The cough is caused by costiveness; the oats will loosen their bowels and the cough will disappear."

Of Thumps or Heaves, A. C. Moore says:

"I have never seen a case but it was preceded by a cough, which was generally worse in the morning, or when the pig first came from its bed. My ordinary remedy is to place a small amount of Tar, the bulk of an egg, well down in the mouth. This can readily be done, by the use of a wooden paddle, and should be done for two or three successive mornings. If the disease does not yield to three doses, I would dissolve one pint of Tar in a gallon of Water, and use one quart as a drench, repeating the dose every morning if required. I do not believe there is a better remedy, though some recommend Tartar Emetic in small doses, mixed with the milk or water given as a drink, and continued from five to ten days. A reliable customer writes me, he has used Tartar-emetic in three cases with perfect success. Another says that two to three spoonsful of Salt, put well down in the throat, is a sure cure.

QUINSY, OR "STRANGLES."

This disease is of frequent occurrence, and rapid in its progress, and generally fatal, and mostly confined to fat hogs, or those fed highly. The first symptoms are: Swelling of glands under the throat, followed by rapid and difficult breathing and difficulty in swallowing; the neck swells and gangrenes, the tongue protrudes from the mouth, and is covered with slaver.

In the beginning of the disease, give an active emetic, such as the following; Potassio-tartrate of Antimony (Tartar-emetic) four grains; Ipecacuanha, six grains; White Hellebore, six grains. Mix and give in food, or throw into the mouth. If the animal will drink anything or eat a little, a purgative powder, consisting of two or three drachms of Castor Oil seeds should be given. When difficulty of breathing is great, apply an active blister over the throat, and give injections frequently. If the animal can swallow, and will drink water, some Sal-ammoniac and Nitre should be dissolved in it.

The recipe below, for Quinsy, is from *Colman's Rural World:*

"When the animal has the disease in a bad form, split the neck on each side of the throat so that it will bleed freely; swab the throat well with Turpentine; make it swallow one or two teaspoonfuls of it; if the subject will drink, this can be given in 'swill' Enough Turpentine poured on corn to make it oily, is a preventive."

NASAL CATARRH, OR "BULL NOSE."

"First symptoms: Unusual discharge from the nose, the inflammation gradually extending to the pharynx, gullet, and larynx. The animal sniffles, coughs some, mucous membrane swells, the nose thickens, and becomes twisted and distorted and ill-shaped, and when exercised a little, the discharge from the nose becomes bloody, or is pure blood. The animal still eats reasonably well, but will not fatten nor grow, but gradually dwindles away, and dies.

"There is little encouragement in trying to cure this, and it is considered by some as being of the same nature as glanders in horses. Animals discovered with the disease should be destroyed, and removed from the farm."

INFLAMMATION OF THE BRAIN, EPILEPSY, OR "BLIND STAGGERS."

This disease frequently attacks swine, especially when changed to rich, abundant food, or exposed to stormy, changeable weather. At first the animal appears dull, stupid, and disinclined to move. The eyes become red and inflamed, the bowels constipated, the pulse hard and quick. In a short time, if not relieved, the animal runs wildly about, usually in a circle, seems blind, will run against objects, the breathing becomes rapid and laborious.

TREATMENT.—Give, at once, a teaspoonful of Calomel, cut a slit in the skin on the head above the eyes, cut it clear to the skull. In this cut put Salt and Pepper to get up a counter-irritation. If this does not succeed, make a liniment as follows: Take a four-ounce vial, into it put one ounce Spirits Turpentine, one ounce Capsicum, one ounce Aqua Ammonia, half ounce Tincture of Arnica, quarter ounce Chloroform; shake well before using, and rub it on, around upper part of the head of the patient, and between the base of the ears and around them.

Professor Law recommends, when a hog is attacked, to dash bucketsful of cold water over the body, and throw into the rectum a purgative injection, composed of six ounces of Sulphate of Soda and one or two teaspoonsfuls of Spirits of Turpentine in ten ounces of Water. Setons saturated with the Turpentine may be inserted under the skin behind the ears; or the back of the neck may be blistered by actively rubbing in the following mixture: Spirits of Turpentine and liquid Ammonia, one ounce of each; powdered Cantharides, two drachms. When it occurs in summer, or in hot weather, its severity can be greatly modified by providing shelter in a shed, where they can be in the shade during the heat of the day; but at the same time a *free circulation* of air should be secured. Water, too, should be constantly within the reach of the animals, and, if possible, a pool of it provided in which they can lie at will.

Dr. Chase says partial recovery will soon occur after securing a free evacuation of the bowels. A teaspoonful of Copperas may be given twice a day, for two weeks, abating the feed somewhat. Also, to never bleed in this disease, as there is a poverty of blood already.

The *North-British Agriculturist* says the disease which is popularly termed staggers, in medical parlance is called epilepsy. It depends usually upon imperfect nutrition of the brain and nervous system. In pigs, as well as in other animals, epilepsy is often hereditary. Frequently it is developed by breeding in-and-in.

APOPLEXY.

Apoplexy only occurs in fat hogs, being caused by a too plethoric condition of the system. It demands prompt treatment, and is indicated by the stupid movements of the animal for perhaps several hours preceding its dropping, as if struck heavily on the head with a sledge-hammer, when the limbs straighten, and but for its heavy breathing, it would be supposed dead.

Dr. Chase says :

"Bleed quickly, by tying a cord tightly around the fore-leg, above the knee, when the brachial vein will be seen to fill up, and may readily be opened with a lancet or sharp pointed knife. The vein is on the inside of the leg, and should be opened about an inch above the knee.

"If possible take a pint and a half of blood, or even more. If this vein does not yield a sufficient amount, some of the veins on the inside of the ear may be opened by turning the ear back and pressing with the thumb firmly on the base. Never cut off an ear or tail for the purpose of drawing blood.

"If the animal recovers from a first attack, at the earliest possible moment give a quarter of a pound of Salts, and repeat it every three hours, until the bowels move freely. Feed lightly for a few days, giving occasional doses of salts, and the probabilities are that it will permanently recover.* * *

"Epilepsy, or blind staggers, is the only disease likely to be confounded with apoplexy."

PARAPLEGIA.

Paralysis of the muscles of the loins in swine is of frequent occurrence, but usually does not seem to interfere with the appetite or general health of the animal.

It is sometimes caused by a severe strain of the back, or blows on the back or loins, producing concussion of the spinal marrow. If such is known to be the cause, cold applications may be tried, for a few days, on the loins and back. If the cause is unknown, and no fever is present in the back, a liniment, composed of equal parts of Cantharides (Spanish Flies), Olive Oil, and Spirits Turpentine, may be applied, or, a seton may be inserted lengthwise under the skin over the loins. The animal should be given comfortable quarters, with freedom from disturbance by others, fed on sloppy, soft food and sour milk, and if costive, frequent injections of warm water should be used.

DIARRHŒA, OR SCOURS.

Young pigs are frequently troubled with diarrhœa. The discharges are of a whitish color, and pigs of sows that have a cold or catarrh are liable to be severely troubled. It rarely attacks old hogs, but is often fatal to young pigs, if not attended to in time. Too much grass or clover, given to a sow when her pigs are quite young, frequently causes this disease. It can generally be checked by shutting the sow up and feeding dry corn for a few days. Skimmed sweet milk fed the sow is also good. If pigs are large enough to eat, give them dry, raw flour, or corn, rye, or wheat, whole.

If too young to eat, a lump of Alum, the size of a walnut, may be dissolved in a quart of water, and a teaspoonful given morning and evening, to pigs a week or so old.

Dr. Mulford says, in the *American Swine and Poultry Journal*:

"Many of our swine breeders in the West sustain considerable loss annually by their pigs dying from the effects of what is commonly called scours, caused by the bad quality of the sow's milk. The disease is more apt to make its appearance when the sow has been fed upon dry corn or musty food. It generally attacks them within one or two days after their birth, and seldom after eight or ten days. I have never failed to cure this disease by giving the sow as much Sulphur of the *third decimal trituration* as will stand on a nickel five-cent piece, once a day. It may be given in a little sweet milk, or upon a small piece of bread, and should be given one hour before feeding. The medicine can be procured of any Homœopathic physician. I have cured many cases with common sulphur, but prefer the above."

Mr. Joseph Harris, in his invaluable work on "The Pig," justly uses the following language:

"The most common complaints of little pigs are diarrhœa and colds. The former is caused by giving the sow improper food, or a too sudden a change of diet, or by irregular feeding, or from want of pure water and fresh air. We once had a few cooked beans that were left in the steam-barrel until they decomposed. They were thrown on to the manure heap, and a sow, which was sucking pigs, ate some of them. Two days afterwards, the whole litter was seized with violent diarrhœa, and one of them died in the course of two or three days. It was the worst case of the kind we ever had, and the diarrhœa continued for four or five days, and was not stopped until we gave the pigs two or three drops of Laudanum each, at night, in some fresh cream, with a teaspoon, and repeated the dose the next morning. This effected a cure, but the pigs did not regain their thrifty growth for a week or ten days. We should add that the sow continued perfectly well, and manifested no symptoms of the complaint. As a general rule, no medicine will be required. Change the food of the mother, and let her go out into the air, but let the little pigs remain in the pen, and see that they are warm and comfortable. The less they are disturbed, and the more they sleep, the sooner will they recover. It is also very important to keep the pen clean and well ventilated. Nothing can be worse than to leave the evacuations in the pen. Scatter some dry earth about the pen to absorb the offensive gases. Let the feeding apartment also be dusted over with dry earth, or soil of any kind that can be obtained, and then scraped, and swept, and washed, and a little dry straw, or chaff, or sawdust, be spread on it, to prevent dampness. Scald the pig troughs with *boiling* water, and make them sweet and clean. Let this be done every day. The attendant should understand that the scours are an evidence of carelessness or negligence."

CONSTIPATION.

If swine are discovered voiding hard, dry dung in compact, ball-like masses, it denotes fever; they require a change to more loosening, cooling diet. Green and any kind of soft, easily digested food is good, and bran mashes prepared with hot water, or if possible, with flax-seed tea are excellent.

In obstinate cases, an ounce of Epsom Salts may be given, in an injection of warm soap suds.

There are few surer indications of something radically wrong in the swine-yard than continued constipation.

EVERSION (TURNING OUT) OF THE RECTUM.

Poorly kept and neglected pigs are liable to protrusion of the rectum, and it may be caused also by straining in parturition, (pig birth), constipation, and diarrhœa.

The protruding part should be emptied, cleaned with warm water, moistened with Laudanum if at hand, gently returned and pushed up with the oiled finger a short distance, inside the anus. In treating this ailment, as well as most others, attention to diet and comfort is all-important.

RHEUMATISM.

SYMPTOMS.—Dullness, languor, or indisposition to move, followed by extreme lameness in one or more limbs, and heat, swelling, or tenderness of a joint, tendon, or group of muscles, the tenderness perhaps shifting from joint to joint.

TREATMENT.—A tablespoonful of Cod-liver Oil should be given to each pig once or twice a day in its food. A larger daily allowance than two tablespoonfuls to pigs three or four months old, while the oil is expensive, does not appear to hasten the cure in like ratio. The cod-liver oil, besides curing the rheumatism, both acute and chronic, also improves the condition wonderfully. Provide well-littered, warm housing, from which the pigs can emerge to the yards at will. Give boiled or steamed food, and sour milk.

PIGS LOSING THEIR TAILS.

Pigs sometimes have their tails frozen, which causes them to drop off, but aside from this cause, it frequently results from an hereditary tendency to a disease of the skin which attacks the young pig at that particular point, the circulation is interfered with, and the member perishes and drops off.

If the disease appears, apply Carbolic Soap to the affected part, or wash clean, and apply Glycerine, Sweet Oil, or a little fresh Lard.

The most effectual preventive is to keep pigs clean, dry, and abundantly nourished.

CANKER OR SORE MOUTH.

Mr. S. M. Shepard, in his excellent book "The Hog in America," thinks this is usually the result of unhealthful milk from the sow or from poison on her teats obtained by contact with poisonous vines or wet grass. He says: "The first symptoms are lumps on the sow's udder, and sometimes sores; next will be noticed blisters on the lip, tongue and mouth of the pig; the tongue and lips become swollen and the roof and sides of the mouth inflamed and covered with deep red or white blister spots. Treatment: Catch the pig and swab its mouth out thoroughly with a solution of carbolic acid and water sufficiently strong to make the flesh upon the arm tingle. Apply with a rag or small piece of sponge tied on a stick. Strong sage tea applied in the same way is good, and in addition blow powdered sulphur through a straw into the pig's mouth. Bathe the sow's teats and udder with a weak solution of carbolic acid, and keep afflicted litters away from other pigs."

INDEX.

Farm Grasses of the United States of America

By WILLIAM JASPER SPILLMAN. A practical treatise on the grass crop, seeding and management of meadows and pastures, description of the best varieties, the seed and its impurities, grasses for special conditions, lawns and lawn grasses, etc., etc. In preparing this volume the author's object has been to present, in connected form, the main facts concerning the grasses grown on American farms. Every phase of the subject is viewed from the farmer's standpoint. Illustrated. 248 pages. 5 x 7 inches. Cloth. $1.0

The Book of Corn

By HERBERT MYRICK, assisted by A. D. SHAMBIA, E. A. BURNETT, ALBERT W. FULTON, B. W. SNOW, and other most capable specialists. A complete treatise on the culture, marketing and uses of maize in America and elsewhere for farmers, dealers and others. Illustrated. 372 pages. 5 x 7 inches. Cloth. $1.50

The Hop—Its Culture and Care, Marketing and Manufacture

By HERBERT MYRICK. A practical handbook on the most approved methods in growing, harvesting, curing and selling hops, and on the use and manufacture of hops. The result of years of research and observation, it is a volume destined to be an authority on this crop for many years to come. It takes up every detail from preparing the soil and laying out the yard, to curing and selling the crop. Every line represents the ripest judgment and experience of experts. Size, 5 x 8; pages, 300; illustrations, nearly 150; bound in cloth and gold; price, postpaid. $1.50

Tobacco Leaf

By J. B. KILLEBREW and HERBERT MYRICK. Its Culture and Cure, Marketing and Manufacture. A practical handbook on the most approved methods in growing, harvesting, curing, packing and selling tobacco, with an account of the operations in every department of tobacco manufacture. The contents of this book are based on actual experiments in field, curing barn, packing house, factory and laboratory. It is the only work of the kind in existence, and is destined to be the standard practical and scientific authority on the whole subject of tobacco for many years. 506 pages and 150 original engravings. 5 x 7 inches. Cloth. $2.00

Bulbs and Tuberous-Rooted Plants

By C. L. Allen. A complete treatise on the history description, methods of propagation and full directions for the successful culture of bulbs in the garden, dwelling and greenhouse. The author of this book has for many years made bulb growing a specialty, and is a recognized authority on their cultivation and management. The cultural directions are plainly stated, practical and to the point. The illustrations which embellish this work have been drawn from nature and have been engraved especially for this book. 312 pages. 5 x 7 inches. Cloth. $1.50

Fumigation Methods

By Willis G. Johnson. A timely up-to-date book on the practical application of the new methods for destroying insects with hydrocyanic acid gas and carbon bisulphid, the most powerful insecticides ever discovered. It is an indispensable book for farmers, fruit growers, nurserymen gardeners, florists, millers, grain dealers, transportation companies, college and experiment station workers, etc. Illustrated. 313 pages. 5 x 7 inches. Cloth. $1.00

Diseases of Swine

By Dr. R. A. Craig, Professor of Veterinary Medicine at the Purdue University. A concise, practical and popular guide to the prevention and treatment of the diseases of swine. With the discussions on each disease are given its causes, symptoms, treatment and means of prevention. Every part of the book impresses the reader with the fact that its writer is thoroughly and practically familiar with all the details upon which he treats. All technical and strictly scientific terms are avoided, so far as feasible, thus making the work at once available to the practical stock raiser as well as to the teacher and student. Illustrated. 5 x 7 inches. 190 pages. Cloth. $0.75

Spraying Crops—Why, When and How

By Clarence M. Weed, D.Sc. The present fourth edition has been rewritten and set throughout to bring it thoroughly up to date, so that it embodies the latest practical information gleaned by fruit growers and experiment station workers. So much new information has come to light since the third edition was published that this is practically a new book, needed by those who have utilized the earlier editions, as well as by fruit growers and farmers generally. Illustrated. 136 pages. 5 x 7 inches. Cloth. $0.50

Successful Fruit Culture

By SAMUEL T. MAYNARD. A practical guide to the cultivation and propagation of Fruits, written from the standpoint of the practical fruit grower who is striving to make his business profitable by growing the best fruit possible and at the least cost. It is up-to-date in every particular, and covers the entire practice of fruit culture, harvesting, storing, marketing, forcing, best varieties, etc., etc. It deals with principles first and with the practice afterwards, as the foundation, principles of plant growth and nourishment must always remain the same, while practice will vary according to the fruit grower's immediate conditions and environments. Illustrated. 265 pages. 5 x 7 inches. Cloth. $1.00

Plums and Plum Culture

By F. A. WAUGH. A complete manual for fruit growers, nurserymen, farmers and gardeners, on all known varieties of plums and their successful management. This book marks an epoch in the horticultural literature of America. It is a complete monograph of the plums cultivated in and indigenous to North America. It will be found indispensable to the scientist seeking the most recent and authoritative information concerning this group, to the nurseryman who wishes to handle his varieties accurately and intelligently, and to the cultivator who would like to grow plums successfully. Illustrated. 391 pages. 5 x 7 inches. Cloth. $1.50

Fruit Harvesting, Storing, Marketing

By F. A. WAUGH. A practical guide to the picking, storing, shipping and marketing of fruit. The principal subjects covered are the fruit market, fruit picking, sorting and packing, the fruit storage, evaporation, canning, statistics of the fruit trade, fruit package laws, commission dealers and dealing, cold storage, etc., etc. No progressive fruit grower can afford to be without this most valuable book. Illustrated. 232 pages. 5 x 7 inches. Cloth. $1.00

Systematic Pomology

By F. A. WAUGH, professor of horticulture and landscape gardening in the Massachusetts agricultural college, formerly of the university of Vermont. This is the first book in the English language which has ever made the attempt at a complete and comprehensive treatment of systematic pomology. It presents clearly and in detail the whole method by which fruits are studied. The book is suitably illustrated. 288 pages. 5 x 7 inches. Cloth. $1.00

Feeding Farm Animals

By Professor THOMAS SHAW. This book is intended alike for the student and the farmer. The author has succeeded in giving in regular and orderly sequence, and in language so simple that a child can understand it, the principles that govern the science and practice of feeding farm animals. Professor Shaw is certainly to be congratulated on the successful manner in which he has accomplished a most difficult task. His book is unquestionably the most practical work which has appeared on the subject of feeding farm animals. Illustrated. 5½ x 8 inches. Upward of 500 pages. Cloth. $2.00

Profitable Dairying

By C. L. PECK. A practical guide to successful dairy management. The treatment of the entire subject is thoroughly practical, being principally a description of the methods practiced by the author. A specially valuable part of this book consists of a minute description of the far-famed model dairy farm of Rev. J. D. Detrich, near Philadelphia, Pa. On the farm of fifteen acres, which twenty years ago could not maintain one horse and two cows, there are now kept twenty-seven dairy cattle, in addition to two horses. All the roughage, litter, bedding, etc., necessary for these animals are grown on these fifteen acres, more than most farmers could accomplish on one hundred acres. Illustrated. 5 x 7 inches. 200 pages. Cloth. $0.75

Practical Dairy Bacteriology

By Dr. H. W. CONN, of Wesleyan University. A complete exposition of important facts concerning the relation of bacteria to various problems related to milk. A book for the classroom, laboratory, factory and farm. Equally useful to the teacher, student, factory man and practical dairyman. Fully illustrated with 83 original pictures. 340 pages. Cloth. 5½ x 8 inches. $1.25

Modern Methods of Testing Milk and Milk Products

By L. L. VANSLYKE. This is a clear and concise discussion of the approved methods of testing milk and milk products. All the questions involved in the various methods of testing milk and cream are handled with rare skill and yet in so plain a manner that they can be fully understood by all. The book should be in the hands of every dairyman, teacher or student. Illustrated. 214 pages. 5 x 7 inches. $0.75

Animal Breeding

By THOMAS SHAW. This book is the most complete and comprehensive work ever published on the subject of which it treats. It is the first book which has systematized the subject of animal breeding. The leading laws which govern this most intricate question the author has boldly defined and authoritatively arranged. The chapters which he has written on the more involved features of the subject, as sex and the relative influence of parents, should go far toward setting at rest the wildly speculative views cherished with reference to these questions. The striking originality in the treatment of the subject is no less conspicuous than the superb order and regular sequence of thought from the beginning to the end of the book. The book is intended to meet the needs of all persons interested in the breeding and rearing of live stock. Illustrated. 405 pages. 5 x 7 inches. Cloth. . . . $1.50

Forage Crops Other Than Grasses

By THOMAS SHAW. How to cultivate, harvest and use them. Indian corn, sorghum, clover, leguminous plants, crops of the brassica genus, the cereals, millet, field roots, etc. Intensely practical and reliable. Illustrated. 287 pages. 5 x 7 inches. Cloth. $1.00

Soiling Crops and the Silo

By THOMAS SHAW. The growing and feeding of all kinds of soiling crops, conditions to which they are adapted, their plan in the rotation, etc. Not a line is repeated from the Forage Crops book. Best methods of building the silo, filling it and feeding ensilage. Illustrated. 364 pages. 5 x 7 inches. Cloth. $1.50

The Study of Breeds

By THOMAS SHAW. Origin, history, distribution, characteristics, adaptability, uses, and standards of excellence of all pedigreed breeds of cattle, sheep and swine in America. The accepted text book in colleges, and the authority for farmers and breeders. Illustrated. 371 pages. 5 x 7 inches. Cloth. $1.50

Clovers and How to Grow Them

By THOMAS SHAW. This is the first book published which treats on the growth, cultivation and treatment of clovers as applicable to all parts of the United States and Canada, and which takes up the entire subject in a systematic way and consecutive sequence. The importance of clover in the economy of the farm is so great that an exhaustive work on this subject will no doubt be welcomed by students in agriculture, as well as by all who are interested in the tilling of the soil. Illustrated. 5 x 7 inches. 337 pages. Cloth. Net . . $1.00

Land Draining

A handbook for farmers on the principles and practice of draining, by MANLY MILES, giving the results of his extended experience in laying tile drains. The directions for the laying out and the construction of tile drains will enable the farmer to avoid the errors of imperfect construction, and the disappointment that must necessarily follow. This manual for practical farmers will also be found convenient for reference in regard to many questions that may arise in crop growing, aside from the special subjects of drainage of which it treats. Illustrated. 200 pages. 5 x 7 inches. Cloth. $1.00

Barn Plans and Outbuildings

Two hundred and fifty-seven illustrations. A most valuable work, full of ideas, hints, suggestions, plans, etc., for the construction of barns and outbuildings, by practical writers. Chapters are devoted to the economic erection and use of barns, grain barns, horse barns, cattle barns, sheep barns, cornhouses, smokehouses, icehouses, pig pens, granaries, etc. There are likewise chapters on birdhouses, doghouses, tool sheds, ventilators, roofs and roofing, doors and fastenings, workshops, poultry houses, manure sheds, barnyards, root pits, etc. 235 pages. 5 x 7 inches. Cloth. $1.00

Irrigation Farming

By LUTE WILCOX. A handbook for the practical application of water in the production of crops. A complete treatise on water supply, canal construction, reservoirs and ponds, pipes for irrigation purposes, flumes and their structure, methods of applying water, irrigation of field crops, the garden, the orchard and vineyard, windmills and pumps, appliances and contrivances. New edition, revised, enlarged and rewritten. Profusely illustrated. Over 500 pages. 5 x 7 inches. Cloth. $2.00

Forest Planting

By H. NICHOLAS JARCHOW, LL. D. A treatise on the care of woodlands and the restoration of the denuded timberlands on plains and mountains. The author has fully described those European methods which have proved to be most useful in maintaining the superb forests of the old world. This experience has been adapted to the different climates and trees of America, full instructions being given for forest planting of our various kinds of soil and subsoil, whether on mountain or valley. Illustrated. 250 pages. 5 x 7 inches. Cloth. $1.50

The Nut Culturist

By ANDREW S. FULLER. A treatise on the propagation, planting and cultivation of nut-bearing trees and shrubs adapted to the climate of the United States, with the scientific and common names of the fruits known in commerce as edible or otherwise useful nuts. Intended to aid the farmer to increase his income without adding to his expenses or labor. Cloth, 12mo. $1.50

Cranberry Culture

By JOSEPH J. WHITE. Contents: Natural history, history of cultivation, choice of location, preparing the ground, planting the vines, management of meadows, flooding, enemies and difficulties overcome, picking, keeping, profit and loss. Illustrated. 132 pages. 5 x 7 inches. Cloth. . . . $1.00

Ornamental Gardening for Americans

By ELIAS A. LONG, landscape architect. A treatise on beautifying homes, rural districts and cemeteries. A plain and practical work with numerous illustrations and instructions so plain that they may be readily followed. Illustrated. 390 pages. 5 x 7 inches. Cloth. $1.50

Grape Culturist

By A. S. FULLER. This is one of the very best of works on the culture of the hardy grapes, with full directions for all departments of propagation, culture, etc., with 150 excellent engravings, illustrating planting, training, grafting, etc. 282 pages. 5 x 7 inches. Cloth. $1.50

Gardening for Young and Old

By JOSEPH HARRIS. A work intended to interest farmers' boys in farm gardening, which means a better and more profitable form of agriculture. The teachings are given in the familiar manner so well known in the author's "Walks and Talks on the Farm." Illustrated. 191 pages. 5 x 7 inches. Cloth. $1.00

Money in the Garden

By P. T. QUINN. The author gives in a plain, practical style instructions on three distinct, although closely connected, branches of gardening—the kitchen garden, market garden and field culture, from successful practical experience for a term of years. Illustrated. 268 pages. 5 x 7 inches. Cloth. $1.00

Made in the USA
Monee, IL
13 September 2026

62976735R00194

The Cornell University Library Digital Collections

This title is part of Cornell University Library's extensive collection of public domain works in subject areas as diverse as American history, English literature, astronomy, food and wine, general engineering, the history of science, home economics, hospitality and travel, human sexuality, labor relations, Native American materials, ornithology, veterinary medicine, and women's studies. Collections already available as reprints from Amazon include titles in New York State historical literature, core historical literature in agriculture, historical mathematics monographs, and materials related to home economics.

One of the leading academic research libraries in the United States, Cornell University Library is a highly valued partner in teaching, research, and learnin at the University. The Library is a leader in digital initiatives, actively buildin its growing network of online resources through local and global partnerships Its outstanding collections—from medieval manuscripts to hip hop and from ancient Chinese texts to comic books—preserve the past and pave the way fo future scholarship. To learn more about Cornell University Library, visit www.library.cornell.edu

Cornell University
Library

9 781112 371080